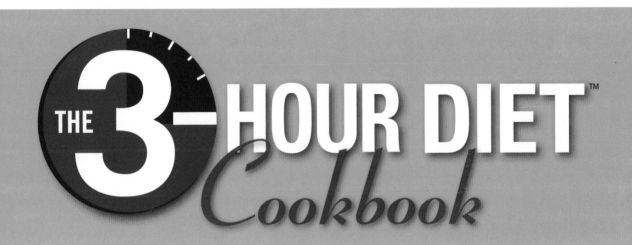

THE 3-HOUR DIET™ Cookbook

PRAISE FOR JORGE CRUISE'S *THE 3-HOUR DIET*™

"Feel like pasta for dinner? Not a problem. Some toast with those eggs? Bring it on. With Jorge's *3-Hour Diet*™, eating great and losing weight has never been this simple."

—Jacqui Stafford, *Shape* magazine

"Combining cutting-edge research with practical how-to, Jorge Cruise's revolutionary approach to eating constitutes a sustainable way to slim down without sacrifice. Jorge offers up powerful kindling that can reignite the motivation of even the most jaded dieter. If you've always wanted a smart, caring weight-loss coach at your disposal 24/7, this book is for you!"

—Carol Brooks, editor in chief, *First for Women* magazine

"Jorge Cruise has identified a fundamental tenet of successful weight loss—that how you eat is just as important as what you eat. His *3-Hour Diet*™ is easy to understand, simple to follow, and specifically designed for those who don't have time to diet. In short, his book is an essential tool for those seeking lifelong weight loss and maintenance."

—Lisa Sanders, MD, Yale University School of Medicine and author of *The Perfect Fit Diet*

"*The 3-Hour Diet*™ offers a simple nutrition prescription: how often and how much to control your hunger, enjoy your food, and improve your health. You can't get much better than that!"

—Leslie Bonci, MPH, RD, LDN, director of sports medicine nutrition, University of Pittsburgh Medical Center, and nutritionist for the Pittsburgh Steelers

"At last, the book to rival the Atkins and South Beach diets is here. If you want to lose weight and keep it off, without giving up any of the food groups, this is the book!"

—John Robbins, author of *Diet for a New America* and *The Food Revolution*

"Jorge has dedicated his life to showing people they can lose weight safely, and this book provides them with the skills to keep the weight off for life. It's a great plan and an inspiring book."

—Kathleen Daelemans, author of *Cooking Thin with Chef Kathleen* and *Getting Thin and Loving Food!*

"Jorge Cruise brings a new dimension to the world of weight loss—empowering and giving you the tools to lose weight by making simple changes in how and when you eat. This technique can help make all the difference."

—Fred Pescatore, MD, author of *The Hamptons Diet* and former associate medical director at the Atkins Center

"Jorge Cruise will keep you looking and feeling your best."

—David Kirsch, author of *The Ultimate New York Body Plan*

"Jorge's *3-Hour Diet*™ offers a sound and practical eating plan. His easy-to-follow guide will help any follower see immediate body transformations with long-lasting results."
—Tammy Lakatos Shames and Lyssie Lakatos, RD, LD, CDN, authors of *Fire Up Your Metabolism*

"Wow! I learned a lot from Jorge's fascinating new book. I can easily see how people who follow the *3-Hour Diet*™ can shed pounds by keeping their fat-burning metabolism revved up."
—Lucy Beale, author of *The Complete Idiot's Guide to Weight Loss*

"An easy alternative to low-carb, high-fat, or other diets that can have harmful side effects."
—Dale Eustace, PhD, professor of cereal technology, Kansas State University

"This simple, easy-to-understand book gives you practical ideas that you can use immediately to lose weight without feeling hungry, without counting calories, and without feeling deprived in any way. I suggest you get one copy for yourself and one for a friend so you can enjoy the process together."
—Christopher Guerriero, founder and chairman of the National Metabolic and Longevity Research Center and author of *Maximize Your Metabolism*

"It's refreshing to hear a popular weight-loss guru pan low-carb and other fad diets and tell people the truth: that they can eat anything in moderation. The plan is nutritionally balanced, smart, and practical. The tone is encouraging and forgiving."
—Janis Jibrin, MS, RD, writer for GoodHousekeeping.com, and author of *The Unofficial Guide to Dieting Safely*

"*The 3-Hour Diet*™ will help millions lose weight and feel great! Eating healthy foods every three hours can help stabilize blood sugar levels, stave off hunger, and melt away unwanted pounds."
—Jay Robb, certified clinical nutritionist, and author of *The Fat Burning Diet*

"Jorge does a great job of creating a straightforward, easy-to-follow eating plan that does not sound like a prison sentence! No restricting carbs, no exotic supplements, and no complex math calculations to make before every meal. *The 3-Hour Diet*™ is easy to read and simple to follow!"
—Harley Pasternak MSc, celebrity trainer, and author of *Five Factor Fitness*

"The goal in life is to get more done in less time, and Jorge Cruise teaches you how to lose the weight you want in a healthy, safe way in *The 3-Hour Diet*™. What could be better? This is a book that can get you to your physical fitness goal in the shortest, easiest, best way ever."
—Mark Victor Hansen, cocreator, #1 *New York Times* bestselling series *Chicken Soup for the Soul*®, coauthor, *The One Minute Millionaire*

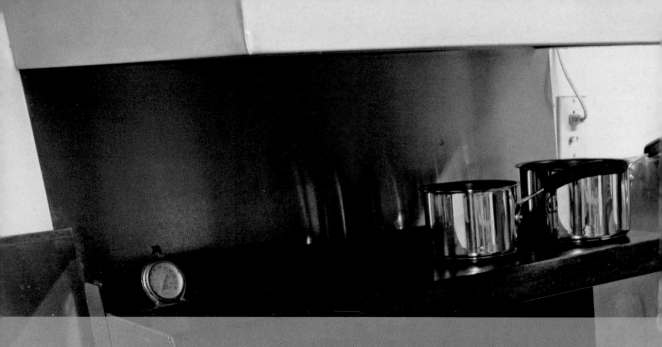

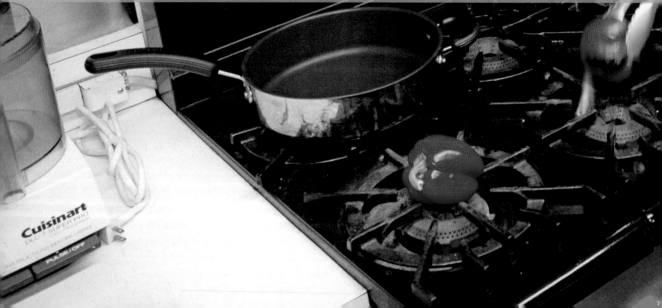

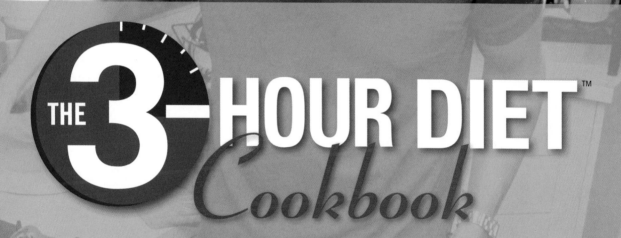

THE 3-HOUR DIET™ Cookbook

LOSE UP TO *10 POUNDS IN THE FIRST 2 WEEKS*

JORGE CRUISE

WM
WILLIAM MORROW
An Imprint of HarperCollinsPublishers

THE 3-HOUR DIET™ COOKBOOK. Copyright © 2007 by JorgeCruise
.com, Inc. All rights reserved. Printed in the United States of
America. No part of this book may be used or reproduced in
any manner whatsoever without written permission except in the
case of brief quotations embodied in critical articles and reviews.
For information address HarperCollins Publishers, 10 East 53rd
Street, New York, NY 10022.

HarperCollins books may be purchased for educational, business,
or sales promotional use. For information please write: Special
Markets Department, HarperCollins Publishers, 10 East 53rd
Street, New York, NY 10022.

Originally published in hardcover in 2007 by Collins, an imprint
of HarperCollins Publishers.

FIRST WILLIAM MORROW PAPERBACK EDITION PUBLISHED 2011.

Designed by Charles Kreloff

Library of Congress Cataloging-in-Publication Data

Cruise, Jorge.

The 3-hour diet cookbook/Jorge Cruise.
p. cm.
Includes index.

ISBN 978-0-06-079318-0
ISBN 978-0-06-111847-0 (pbk.)

1. Reducing diets—Recipes. I. Title.

RM222.2.C769   2007
613.2'5—dc22   2006051163

11 12 13 14 15 ❖/RRD 10 9 8 7 6 5 4

This book is dedicated to Jane Friedman. Thank you for your guidance, friendship, and vision. You have made the 3-Hour Diet™ revolution a reality.

And to Lisa Sharkey, an incredible woman who believed in me from the very start.

Thank you to my colleagues for their extraordinary support and belief throughout the years:

Mike & Rick Anderson
Edward Ash-Miliby
Tyra Banks
Bruce Barlean
Jade Beutler
George Bick
Bonnie Block
Liz Brody
Bobbi Brown
Cathy Chermol
Dusty Cohen
Katie Couric
Chris Cuomo
Jack Curry
Margit Detweiler
Mary Doherty

Hilary Estey-Mcloughlin
Natalie Farage
Joe Fusco
Bill Geddie
Terry Goodman
Lisa
   Gregorisch-Dempsey
Michelle Hatty
Kathy Huck
David Katz, MD
Ellen Levine
Shelby Meizlik
Joanna Powell
Sheila Rosenbaum
John Redmann
Al Roker

Janet Rolle
Amy Rosenblum
Arnold Schwarzenegger
  & Maria Shriver
Roni Selig
Jacqui Stafford
Martha Stewart
Suzanne Somers and
   Alan Hamel
Joe Tessitore
David Thomsen
Reid Tracy
Bob Tuschman
Mark Victor
Barbara Walters
Bob Wietrak

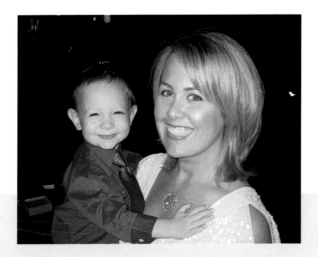

Special thanks to

To my beautiful wife, Heather. She is the single most important woman who has helped me become the man I am today. Thank you for bringing so much to my life. I am so grateful I have you in my life, doll.

Then a big thank you to my two sons: Parker and baby Owen. You both have made my life complete. You bring new joy, happiness, and excitement to me every day. I love you with all my heart.

To my team at my office who support my dream and vision of empowering America with the 3HourDiet.com center. Thanks to Trixie Kennedy, Kathy Thomas, Chad Wagner, Oliver Stephenson, Jared Davis, and Gretchen Lees.

A very special thank you to Auriana Albert, my culinary assistant, for helping me refine the recipes in this book.

To my dear friend Emeril Lagasse for all his extraordinary support with this cookbook. Thank you for having me as a guest on your show and for the very kind endorsement. And an additional thank you to your amazing team: Karen Katz, Charissa Cabot, Suzanne Cornelius, Mara Warner, and Tony Cruz.

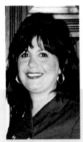

Marlisa Brown

And a special acknowledgment to Marlisa Brown, a dear friend and nutritional/culinary guru who helped me develop certain recipes, providing me with recipe refinements and magic. Marlisa is an independent nutrition/culinary expert, Registered Dietician, chef, and Certified Diabetes Educator of Total Wellness, Inc. (www.TWellness.net).

I'd also like to thank Dr. Jennifer Lovejoy of Bastyr University (www.bastyr.edu) for her recipe contributions and knowledge of diet and wellness. Many of the recipes in this book were developed in association with the School of Nutrition and Exercise Science at Bastyr University: at the heart of natural medicine.

I want to thank Ed Ouellette for his beautiful cover and interior photographs. Thank you to Natalie Ritenour for her lovely candid pictures. And a big thank you to Ray Kau at Whole Foods Market Hillcrest for allowing us to use their location for candid shots.

Thank you to Denise Vivaldo and her incredibly talented team of stylists at FoodFanatics.net: Cindie Flannigan, Beth Fortune, Jennifer Story, and Paty Winters.

And a big thank you to all my 3HourDiet.com online clients for their feedback on these recipes. Your comments and feedback helped give this cookbook five stars!

CONTENTS

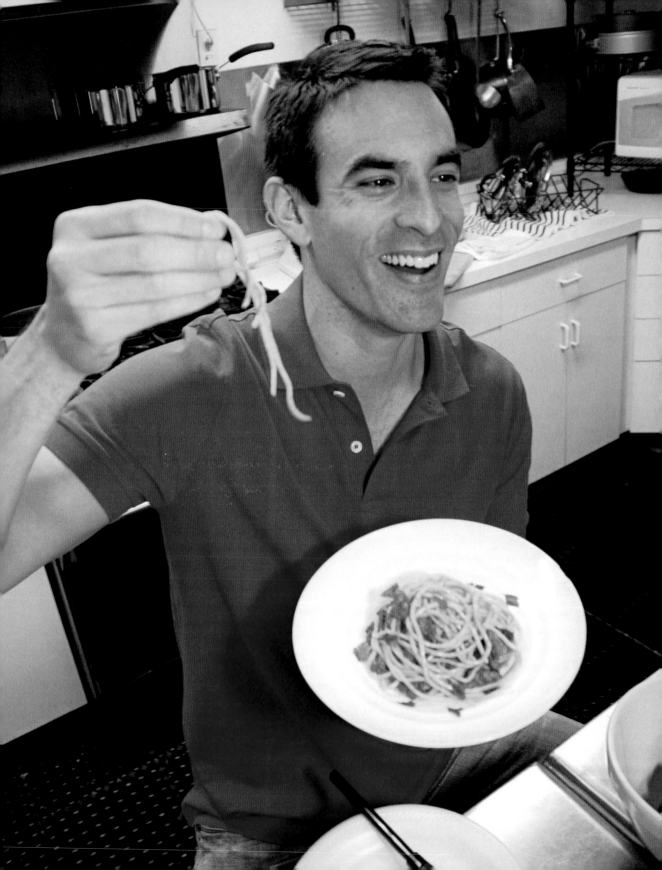

INTRODUCTION

From the desk of Jorge Cruise

Dear Friend,

The biggest mistake you can make when trying to lose weight is to skip meals. When you skip meals throughout the day your blood sugar plummets, causing you to overeat. And when you overeat, you gain weight.

When you eat the *right foods* every three hours you will not feel hungry. Keeping your blood sugar level stable is the secret. The bottom line is that by eating the right foods every three hours, you will be in control of your appetite and *lose up to 10 pounds in 2 weeks*!

What are the right foods? The answer is in this cookbook. There are more than 200 ready-in-minutes meals that are *small in calories, but big in taste*. They are truly irresistible. And the best news is that none of your favorite foods will be off-limits—from pizza to burgers to pasta and much more. It's all here.

So here's my challenge to you: start to use this cookbook today and get ready to lose up to 10 pounds in the first two weeks. Your whole outlook on life will improve when you start noticing how much more energy you have, how much better your clothes fit, and how much better you look. Your self-confidence will skyrocket. Visualize how great it will feel to be happy, healthy, and proud of yourself and your appearance.

So, let's get started!

Your coach,

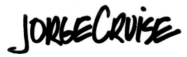

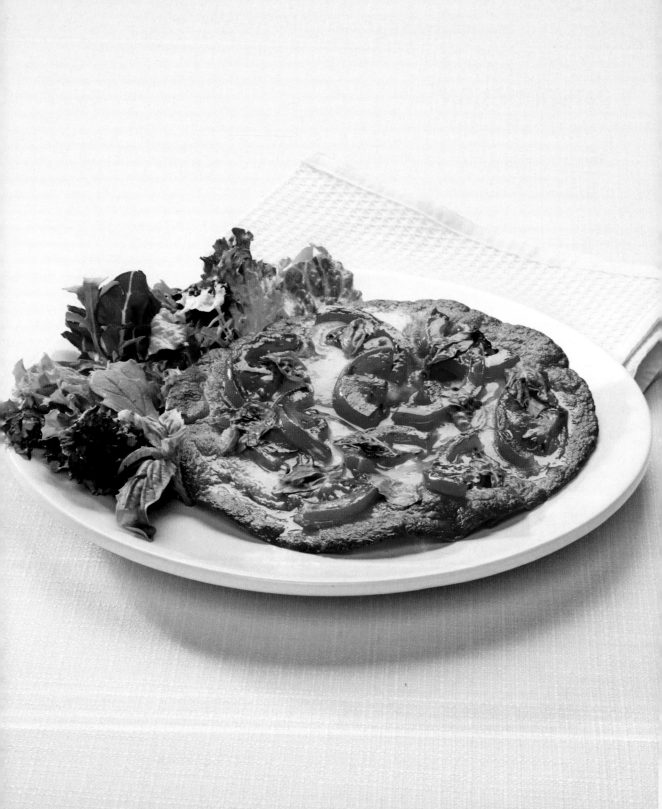

Part 1
IT'S ALL ABOUT TIMING

Chapter 1
WHAT IS THE 3-HOUR DIET™?

As I stated in the introduction, the biggest mistake you can make when you're trying to lose weight is to skip meals, because you'll lose control of your appetite and overeat. *And* it causes your metabolism to slow down because your body will consume precious fat-burning lean muscle.

But when you eat the *right foods* every three hours, you literally change your body's biochemistry, and you gain instant control over your appetite—especially at night. Yes, that is one of the most powerful benefits of our diet. You will gain control of your eating and the weight will quickly come off and stay off. So keep reading, because your waistline will never be the same.

A Revolution in Nutrition

One of my most memorable clients, Victoria, is a busy thirty-six-year-old mother of a teenager. She lost 20 pounds on the 3-Hour Diet™. According to Victoria: "Before I ran across this diet, I was depressed. Our family ate whenever we could, whatever we could. Because we are busy people, we frequently ate one or two meals a day: huge, unhealthy meals. But, this plan makes sense. I have a way of life that keeps me healthy and optimistic."

JORGE CRUISE
LOST 34 POUNDS!

Height:	6' 1"
Age:	35
Starting weight:	219 lbs.
Current weight:	185 lbs.
About me:	Married to my beautiful wife, Heather, with my sons, Parker and Owen

"I grew up a fat kid. I was so chubby that my mom used to call me 'el rey' (the king) in Spanish. However, the nicknames that I heard at school were less endearing— 'lard-ass' and 'fatso.'

"When I was a teenager, two life-altering events forced me to take stock of my weight and my health—my appendix burst and my dad was diagnosed with prostate cancer. I resolved to focus on improving my health and fitness.

"I created this plan—the 3-Hour Diet™—because none of the existing plans helped control my hunger. I also incorporated just a few minutes each day of strength training to build muscle and burn more fat. My eating and exercise plan was so simple and easy that I was able to sustain it, even being married, being a dad with two active boys, and running the 3HourDiet.com weight control center."

JORGE'S SECRETS TO SUCCESS

• Always start your day with a plan! I like to organize my meals at least the night before using the meal planner on our Web site, 3HourDiet.com. It's much easier to stick to your weight loss goals when you have a solid printed plan.

• Remind yourself to eat every three hours. If you're like me, then your day often gets so hectic that you forget to eat! Get a watch with a timer on it or, as a member of our Web site, you can download our special timer from 3HourDiet.com, to remind yourself of your next meal.

• Have snacks on hand. You'll be less likely to cheat on your diet when you keep 100-calorie snacks with you at all times. My favorite snack is raw almonds—twelve of them; they're convenient, delicious, and incredibly good for you.

Source: 3HourDiet.com

Victoria is not alone in her opinion. The 3-Hour Diet™ is truly a revolution in nutrition. It introduces the concept of *timing*—the fact that *when* you eat is just as important as *what* you eat. The 3-Hour Diet™ is what I call *Time-Based Nutrition*. When you eat the right foods at the right times, you will see fat disappear every week and not return. When you eat at the wrong times, you slow down your metabolism and gain weight over the long term.

Why does eating every three hours have such a beneficial impact on your body? How does it work? I will now share with you all the reasons why this diet is so effective and some of the scientific research that backs up this nutritional revolution.

Naturally Suppresses the Appetite

Many people think that eating every three hours will cause them to eat more throughout the day, which will make them gain weight. In fact, the opposite is true.

When you eat every three hours, you keep your blood sugar level stable, which automatically suppresses your appetite. Research has proven that people who eat small, frequent meals binge less often and have fewer cravings than people who eat large, sporadic meals.

One study conducted in the Netherlands found that obese women who ate small, frequent meals had higher levels of leptin hormones than obese women who ate fewer, larger meals. Leptin is a hormone produced by fat cells that plays a major role in suppressing appetite. **The bottom line: the study found that the women who ate more frequently felt less hungry and had fewer cravings throughout the day.**

Turns off the Starvation Protection Mechanism

The number one reason why I tell clients to eat every three hours is to turn off the starvation protection mechanism (SPM). What is the SPM? It's the body's natural defense against starvation. **When you go more than three hours without eating, the SPM is triggered and your body preserves fat and consumes precious fat-burning lean muscle.** But when the SPM is turned off, the body burns fat and preserves muscle.

You see, thousands of years ago, our ancestors adapted to a "feast or famine" existence. When conditions were ideal, people feasted on meat, foliage, nuts, berries, and other foods. At other times, however, when food was scarce, they went days and sometimes weeks without eating. To survive, their bodies developed a way to conserve fat—the body's most valuable, calorie-rich tissue—during famine. When it sensed that food was scarce, the body slowed down the metabolism to preserve fat. This ensured survival by holding on to tissue that could sustain the body through times of famine.

Many studies support the 3-Hour Diet™ concept of eating every three hours to lose fat. Here is a small sample of what research has found:

- In a study published in the *British Journal of Nutrition*, weight loss participants who ate frequent meals preserved considerably more lean muscle tissue than participants who ate fewer daily meals but consumed the same number of calories.

- Scandinavian researchers arrived at similar results when they tested two diets on a group of athletes who were trying to lose weight. Although all of them lost the same amount of weight, the participants who ate fewer meals lost mostly lean muscle tissue, whereas the ones who ate more frequent meals lost almost all fat tissue.

- One of my favorite clinical trials was reported in the *Journal of Human Clinical Nutrition*: weight loss increased and the loss of lean muscle was minimized in a group of obese women who ate every three hours versus another group of obese women who ate every six hours.

Increases Basal Metabolic Rate

When you spread your calories out throughout the day, your body receives calories as it needs them. **Your cells can then quickly take up blood sugar as it becomes available and burn it for energy.** When you eat fewer, larger meals, your body cannot burn as many calories as you consume and stores those excess calories as fat. As a result, you gain weight, even though you may be eating the same number of calories throughout the day.

Increases Energy Level

Most people are familiar with a slump in energy in the late afternoon. Usually this slump results from going too long without food. When you go too long without eating, your blood sugar level drops and your energy plummets. It's hard to concentrate, and all you want to do is nap. **However, when you eat every three hours, you keep your blood sugar level stable and provide a continuous supply of energy to your brain and muscles.**

Reduces the Belly-bulging Hormone Cortisol

Cortisol is a stress-induced hormone, and high levels of cortisol are closely associated with excess abdominal fat. A study conducted by the Department of Nutritional Sciences in Toronto, Canada, showed that eating every three hours helped reduce levels of cortisol. **The study found that participants who ate frequent small meals, as opposed to three large meals that contained the same number of calories, reduced their cortisol levels by more than 17 percent.** If these participants could be so successful in only two weeks, imagine what a lifetime of three-hour eating could do for you!

Basic Rules for the 3-Hour Diet™

So, now you know how eating every three hours can improve your health and help you lose weight. But how do you incorporate this plan into your busy life? Well, there are **three simple rules** to follow on the 3-Hour Diet™: 1) eat your first meal within one hour of waking up, 2) eat every three hours, and 3) stay flexible. That's it. And with this book all the calorie counting has been done for you, so you don't have to wonder if you're eating too much or not enough. It couldn't be simpler. Let's take a look at the rules that will ensure that you reach your weight loss goals.

Eat Within One Hour of Rising

You must eat your first meal within one hour of rising. As you sleep, your body isn't getting any food and consequently turns down your metabolism. Therefore, it's important to kick-start your metabolism back into high gear as soon as possible. If you don't eat within one hour of waking, your body will protect its most valuable, calorie-rich tissue that it needs to survive during a famine—body fat—and cannibalize muscle instead of fatty tissue. That's why it's so important to eat breakfast within one hour of rising every morning. If you skip breakfast, you just end up sabotaging your diet efforts.

Eat Every Three Hours

As we explained earlier, you must eat every three hours to succeed on the 3-Hour Diet™. Eating every three hours keeps your blood sugar level stable, which helps you control your appetite. When your appetite is under control, you won't overeat at vulnerable times, such as in the evening, and you won't gain weight. When you control your appetite, you control your weight.

I suggest that you start out with breakfast every day at 7 a.m., have a snack at 10 a.m., eat lunch at 1 p.m., have another snack at 4 p.m., and eat dinner at 7 p.m. You can finish your day with a treat, either with dinner or anytime within the next three hours before bed. This is an ideal eating schedule, and I strongly recommend that you follow this pattern.

Stay Flexible

In today's hectic world, not everyone can follow the same daily schedule. The 3-Hour Diet™ is designed to bend with unique schedules to ensure *stress-free dieting* by allowing you to move certain meals and snacks around. The following are a couple of sample diet plans that can help you configure the 3-Hour Diet™ to your personal schedule.

For the Early Bird

4 a.m.:   Breakfast
7 a.m.:   Snack
10 a.m.:   Lunch
1 p.m.:   Snack
4 p.m.:   Dinner
7 p.m.:   Treat

For the Late Riser

10 a.m.:   Breakfast
1 p.m.:   Lunch
4 p.m.:   Snack
7 p.m.:   Dinner
9 p.m.:   Treat and snack

For the Very Late Riser

Noon: Lunch
3 p.m.:   Snack
6 p.m.:   Late lunch (early dinner) AND snack
9 p.m.:   Dinner AND treat

Although it's important to stay on schedule with your three-hour eating, real-world obstacles sometimes get in the way. The solution? Stay flexible. As long as you keep close to the three-hour window, you'll be fine. Ideally, don't allow more than an extra thirty minutes to pass before your next meal or snack.

The Importance of Water

No weight loss guide would be complete without including a discussion of the importance of drinking water. Drinking a lot of water is essential to successful weight loss. More than half of your body is made up of water, and water helps keep nearly all of your body functions working properly. In addition, since it's filling and calorie-free, drinking water staves off hunger and keeps you from overeating.

WATER: HOW TO MAKE IT TASTE GREAT

In helping my online clients lose weight, I've discovered that many people simply don't like water. They don't like the way it tastes. In our culture of sugary sodas, fruit juice drinks, and other supersweet beverages, people are conditioned to seek a more intensely flavored beverage than water. This is problematic, because most sweet drinks are laden with high-calorie sugar and high-fructose corn syrup, which are devastating America's waistlines.

So, what we need is a way to make water taste better so more people will drink it. This is easier than you think, and you don't need to add sugary substances to do that. Here are some suggestions for how to improve the way water tastes to encourage you to drink it instead of sodas or juice:

1. Most tap water leaves a chemical aftertaste. So, for cleaner tasting water you should switch to bottled water.

2. Many spas offer water flavored with citrus fruits, like lemon, lime, and orange. Re-create this spa experience at home by filling a pitcher with ice water and dropping in a few thin slices of the fruit of your choice.

3. Sparkling water, such as Perrier®, is convenient, flavorful, and filling, because of the carbonation. Add a squeeze of lemon or lime to vary the flavor.

4. Various naturally flavored waters have made an appearance on the market, such as Propel® Fitness Water by the folks who make Gatorade®. Propel® Fitness water comes in lots of delicious flavors, like melon, peach, grape, lemon, berry, black cherry, kiwi strawberry, mixed berry, and mandarin orange. These beverages are delicious, all-natural, low-calorie, and convenient.

These are just a few options for ways to get more water in your diet. People often mistake thirst for hunger, so the next time you feel the urge to snack, try chugging a glass of lemon-flavored water instead. Chances are, it will take care of your craving.

Drinking a lot of water can also increase your metabolism by boosting your oxygen levels. One German study discovered that drinking one 16-ounce glass of water boosts metabolism by 30 percent within forty minutes and keeps the metabolism elevated for more than an hour.

Finally, drinking a lot of water will increase your energy level. When you're dehydrated, you feel tired, because your heart has to work harder to pump your thickened blood throughout your body. As a result, your organs and muscles don't get all the nutrients they need as quickly as they should.

To make sure that you get enough water, keep an eye on your urine. It should be light-colored or clear. If it's dark or strong-smelling, you need to drink more. Other signs of dehydration include fatigue, headaches, and difficulty concentrating. Don't rely on feeling thirsty to tell you when you need more water; if you're thirsty, you're already dehydrated.

Here are two ways to ensure that you drink enough water:

- Drink a glass of water first thing in the morning. You may discover that you no longer need a morning cup of coffee. Dehydration is a major reason why many people are tired in the morning.

- Drink a glass of water before every meal. The body's signal for thirst is often misinterpreted as the signal for hunger. Drinking a glass of water will keep you in control of your appetite and ensure that you stick with the portions on your 3-Hour Plate™ (see sidebar on p.16).

So, now you know what the 3-Hour Diet™ is all about and how you can use it to gain control of your weight and health. Remember, the 3-Hour Diet™ is based on the premise that skipping meals is devastating to your weight loss success. Not eating causes your blood sugar level to drop, which makes you hungry. Being hungry will make you lose control of your appetite and overeat at mealtimes. To avoid overeating, emotional eating, or eating too-large portions, utilize the principles of the 3-Hour Diet™ and feed your body the right foods every three hours.

I challenge you to live the 3-Hour Diet™ and see how this plan will help you reach your goal weight. Sign the 3-Hour Diet™ Success Contract and put it in plain view on your refrigerator. Each time you seek food when your body doesn't need it, you'll be reminded of your commitment and your future body, and temptation will no longer be a problem.

MY 3-HOUR DIET SUCCESS CONTRACT

Filling out this contract will help keep you accountable to your goals. Make three copies and give them to three trusted friends who will support and motivate you in your journey to success.

Name: _____

Today's date: _____

I am going to weigh this many pounds: _____

By this date: _____

_____

Signature

Photocopy this contract and place on your refrigerator. Join 3-HourDiet.com for support and to stay accountable.

MICHELE TROMBLEY
LOST 86 POUNDS!

Height:	5' 7½"
Age:	40
Starting weight:	207 lbs.
Current weight:	121 lbs.
About Michele:	Married 17 years, with twins (a boy and a girl); works part-time at an elementary school.

"After a long vacation in Florida with my husband and thirteen-year-old twins, I could no longer look at myself in a photo, let alone in a mirror. One morning, I woke up to my favorite show, *Good Morning America*, and there was Jorge talking with Diane Sawyer.

"I wanted a healthy eating plan, because I knew from taking the dieting plunge so many times that I did not want to deprive myself or I would quit, as I always did.

"I started eating the way Jorge recommended. Looking at my dinner plate in a whole new way seemed too easy, but I loved it! That first week, I was feeling better than I had felt in years, and I lost 7 pounds! I reached my goal weight on my birthday, and I feel younger and better than ever."

MICHELE'S SECRETS TO SUCCESS

- Prioritize everything that is important, either in your head or on a calendar or piece of paper.

- Get ready for your next day the night before. Have lunches and dinners decided for the week, so that when you go shopping, you only get the things you need.

- Keep it healthy—don't deprive yourself!

Source: 3HourDiet.com

RONIKA VAUGHN
LOST 40 POUNDS!

Height:	5' 3"
Age:	22
Starting weight:	155 lbs.
Current weight:	115 lbs.
About Ronika:	Kentucky native and schoolteacher

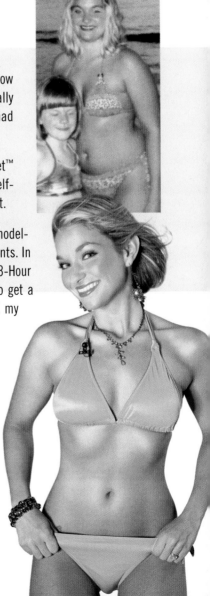

"Before using the 3-Hour Diet™ I was very unhappy with my body and had very low self-esteem. My energy level had decreased to a point where I had become totally inactive. I was suffering physically and emotionally by being overweight. I knew I had to get in charge of my health, so I chose to do the 3-Hour Diet™.

"As soon as I started the plan, I saw immediate results. Since using The 3-Hour Diet™ I have gone from 155 to 115—I lost 40 pounds and changed my life entirely. My self-confidence grew day after day, and before I knew it I had achieved my goal weight.

"By reaching my goal, I have had many opportunities with beauty pageants and modeling. After I lost the weight, I started entering swimsuit contests and beauty pageants. In the near future, I hope to further my modeling/acting career. I plan to stay on the 3-Hour Diet™ for the rest of my life to stay fit and healthy. If I ever get lucky enough to get a modeling contract, it will be a direct result of The 3-Hour Diet™; it has changed my life dramatically.

RONIKA'S SECRETS TO SUCCESS

• Always write grocery lists before shopping. I like to organize mine by different food groups to make sure that I shop efficiently.

• When you're cooking, lay out everything you need before you start—pots, pans, protein, veggies, knives, etc. That way you don't waste time looking for what you need in the middle of preparing a meal.

• With a Crock-Pot® and George Foreman® Grill, you'll be able to make tasty food quickly and healthfully!

Source: 3HourDiet.com

Chapter 2
GETTING YOURSELF OUTFITTED

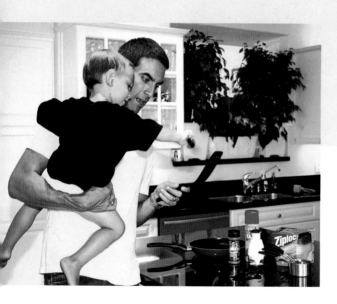

Many of my clients tell me that they don't like to cook. Why? They have NO time. Face it, most of us live such busy lives between school, work, children, and marriages that we just can't fit a half hour to an hour of cooking into each day.

That's why I put together this chapter. The goal is to share with you the tools you need to cook delicious, healthy meals in just minutes. In order to succeed at losing weight, you must be able to cook efficiently and quickly so that dieting can easily fit into your lifestyle. If you outfit your kitchen according to the following guidelines, you will have fresh, healthy food at all times so you can continue your path through the 3-Hour Diet™ to success.

I believe that you only need *seven* tools in your kitchen to prepare delicious, wholesome, weight-controlling meals in no time. These items will help you season food perfectly, so that each item is not only healthy, but also appetizing and a pleasure to eat. In addition, these items make preparing food so easy and convenient that they will encourage you to have

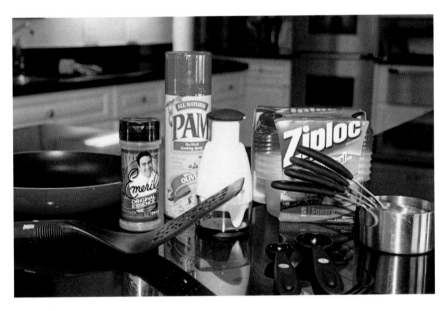

healthy food on hand at all times. Plus, 3-Hour Diet™ recipes were formulated to take no more than ten minutes of cooking time. These items will help you prepare these recipes quickly, so that you have more time in your day to do the things you really enjoy.

The following seven items are indispensable in my kitchen, and I believe you will find them just as necessary in yours.

All Natural PAM® Extra Virgin Olive Oil Spray (www.pamforyou.com)

Extra virgin olive oil contains one of the healthiest kind of fats—monounsaturated fats. Monounsaturated fats lower your risk of developing coronary artery disease by reducing blood-cholesterol levels. In addition, extra virgin olive oil contains large amounts of antioxidants, which are thought to reduce the risk of several types of cancer.

Despite these amazing health benefits of olive oil, we must remember that it is a pure fat, and therefore is high in calories. Using an aerosol or pump spray, such as All Natural PAM® Extra Virgin Olive Oil, drastically reduces the amount of oil you need to keep your food from sticking to your pan. Less fat equals fewer calories, which equals greater weight control.

HOW TO EAT OUT:
THE 3-HOUR PLATE™

One of the best aspects of the 3-Hour Diet™ is that you will never have to ban foods, count calories, or deprive yourself of your favorite foods. Fad diets—diets that restrict certain food groups—inevitably fail, because those forbidden foods are so enticing that you eventually cheat and sabotage your success. There's no cheating on the 3-Hour Diet™, because no foods are taboo! I like to say, "There's no bad food, only bad portions."

What do you do if you are eating out? Well, all you have to do is visualize my 3-Hour Plate™ and you will know exactly what and how much to eat. For any breakfast, lunch, or dinner, use a standard 9-inch plate and fill half of it with vegetables or fruit (about the size of three DVD cases). Then, divide the other half of the plate into two parts and fill the remainder of the plate with carbohydrates the size of a Rubik's Cube, protein the equivalent of a deck of playing cards, and a teaspoon of fat about the size of a water bottle cap. If you're still hungry after finishing the plate, you can add another pile of vegetables or fruit, about the size of three DVD cases. It really is that simple!

If you utilize the visual 3-Hour Plate™ while dining out, you'll never struggle with weight control again. If you want access to my approved on-the-go 3-Hour Diet™ lists, then be sure to join 3HourDiet.com—and eating out will be even easier. Once you are a member, you will have access to our fast food, frozen food, and even bars/shakes lists.

Emeril's Essence® Spices—Original, Bayou Blast, Bam It! Salad Seasoning, and Garlic Parmesan (www.emerils.com)

Emeril's Essence® Spices are a great way to add more flavor to any 3-Hour Diet™ meal without adding calories. They are delectable, dried spice mixes that can be added to chicken, fish, vegetables, or anything that could use an added punch or "BAM!" as Emeril would say. All this fantastic flavor with no fat or calories? You just can't beat it.

GladWare® (www.glad.com)

One of the biggest roadblocks to healthy eating and sustained weight control is convenience. That's where GladWare® comes into play. I love these handy containers. They're inexpensive, durable, dishwasher- and microwave-safe, and stackable, so they'll fit in your cabinet or refrigerator. You can store leftovers, cut vegetables, diced fruit, salads, and soups to take on the go. These useful storage containers are essential in any busy household.

Measuring Cups and Spoons

Measuring ingredients accurately is an important factor in losing weight and keeping it off. Many people try to "eyeball" measurements and fail to recognize how drastically off they are. Inaccurate measuring results in larger portions of fat, sugar, or other ingredients, and people end up eating far more calories than they realize. Measuring is a good habit to get in to.

Spatula

A soft, silicone-coated spatula is essential to preparing delicious, healthy, hot foods in your kitchen. A spatula makes flipping eggs, turning chicken or burger patties, and sautéing a breeze, even for the reluctant or novice cook. Choose a silicone- or rubber-coated spatula instead of a metal spatula to avoid scratching your pans. As an added benefit, silicone-coated utensils won't melt at high-cooking temperatures, unlike plastic utensils.

Nonstick Skillet

The nonstick skillet is every dieter's best friend. Its durable, slick Teflon® coating doesn't need any added fat to prevent your food from sticking. One quick spray of PAM® is all you need to enhance your food's texture and flavor. These pans are easy on cleanup, too—a quick swipe with a soft sponge is usually all you need.

OXO® Chopper (www.oxo.com)

The OXO Chopper is a great tool for the dieter who wants to add fresh ingredients to entrees without having to fumble with a large knife. Its sharp blade is encased in a plastic column, so it's safe even for children to use. At the touch of a plunger, the chopper quickly and safely reduces garlic cloves, onions, tomatoes, or fresh herbs to a perfect mince, ready to add to salads, casseroles, or sauces. This tool is ideal for busy homes who want fresh, tasty meals in a minimum amount of time.

So, there you have the *seven* items that I believe are essential to losing weight healthfully and keeping it off forever. These tools will make your life much easier in the kitchen. But what about stocking your kitchen pantry? Well, read on, because it's not as complicated as you might think.

Fresh, Frozen, or Canned?

My clients frequently ask me how to choose between fresh, frozen, or canned foods. There's a bewildering array of products on the market, and they want to know how to choose food that fits the 3-Hour Diet™ guidelines. Well, I tell them that the 3-Hour Diet™ is primarily concerned with calories, timing, and convenience. So, as long as you're following your three-hour eating schedule and eating the proper number of calories, it doesn't matter how you consume your fruits and veggies.

Having said that, I do think that fresh produce is usually superior to frozen or canned in both nutrition and flavor. However, it can be inconvenient and time-consuming to prep fruits and vegetables for every meal.

Who has time to wash, dry, and tear lettuce for salads every day? Not me. Because I'm so busy, I turn to convenience foods whenever I have to. But which do I choose among the countless options in modern supermarkets? Here's a brief rundown of when to use fresh, frozen, and canned produce as well as a guide to choosing prepared foods.

Fresh

Fresh produce is best when: 1) it's allowed to ripen on its own, 2) only a little time passes between picking and serving, and 3) it undergoes minimal cooking. The less time that passes between picking and eating, the more nutrients the produce will retain. So, look for fresh fruits and vegetables at local farmers' markets or, if you can, grow your own in a garden.

Fresh fruits and veggies are best in their whole, unadulterated state; for example, a mixed green salad or grilled vegetables are best with fresh instead of frozen or canned alternatives. They're delicious on their own, and minimal cooking will allow the fresh, natural flavor to shine through.

Many grocery stores now carry fresh fruits and vegetables that have been prepped for you, such as prewashed, bagged salad mixes; cut-up fruit salads; sliced carrots, celery, onions, and bell peppers. Look for these conveniences to help you get fresh produce to the table more often.

My clients often ask whether they should buy organic fruits and veggies. Well, I say that organic is great . . . if you can afford it. Organic simply means that the food was produced without the use of synthetic chemicals, like pesticides or, in the case of animal products, growth hormones. It's not necessary to eat organic to lose weight, and I always urge my clients to lean toward whatever is most convenient for them—if it's not convenient, it's hard to stick with in the long term. However, if you have access to organic products and can afford them, then by all means, eat organic.

Frozen

Frozen produce is second best to fresh. In fact, frozen can sometimes be more nutritious than fresh. You see, veggies and fruit are picked at their peak of ripeness and quickly frozen before being packaged and shipped, which captures all the nutrients in their mature state. Fresh produce, on the other hand, is usually picked underripe, and then boxed and shipped, sometimes for several weeks, across the country. The produce loses a lot of its nutrients and freshness during those weeks. So, if you don't have access to a farmers' market or don't know how fresh the veggies at your local supermarket are, it might be more nutritious to buy frozen.

Frozen veggies are great in cooked items, such as casseroles or stir-fries. Plus, they're convenient, because a lot of them are chopped and sliced for you already. They also come in a variety of mixes, such as fajita, stir-fry, and other veggie mixes.

Canned

Canned produce is the least nutritious of the three options, but it's not wholly without nutritional value. The canning factories are usually within a few miles of where the food was harvested, which reduces the amount of processing time, and therefore minimizes nutrient loss, between picking and processing. Foods are first blanched—cooked quickly in boiling water or steam—and then packed in cans or jars. Because of this cooking process, canned foods aren't as visually appealing as fresh, but it's better to eat canned fruits and veggies than none at all.

One thing to keep in mind when purchasing canned products is what the foods are canned in. Canned veggies, for example, are often packed in sodium-saturated liquid, which can wreak havoc on your blood pressure. Canned fruits are often packed in heavy sugar syrup, which add tons of calories. Instead of these unhealthy options, look for low-sodium canned veggies and fruits canned in juice. Not only will these items help you keep your calories in check, but they'll also taste more like the real thing.

Prepared Items

Several of the recipes in this book call for prepared foods, such as marinara sauce, salad dressings, barbecue sauce, or cooked chicken. If you have the time and inclination to make your own sauces and dressings,

SECRETS TO ENSURING YOUR SUCCESS
STAY ORGANIZED

Your 3-Hour Timeline™ will be your secret weapon in staying organized with your weight loss plan. Every day, on a sheet of paper, draw a long vertical line with an arrow pointing down. This line will represent your day. Draw six horizontal lines through the vertical line to represent each meal, snack, and treat for the day.

Next, on the far left, indicate the time you choose to eat each meal, snack, and treat. Finally, on the right, add the foods you plan to eat that day. Don't forget to include eight circles on the bottom to represent your eight glasses of water. It's that simple! If you want to try our official online meal planner visit 3HourDiet.com and see how easy staying organized can be.

7 AM	Breakfast	-Lean Pocket -½ cup cottage cheese + fruit
10 AM	Snack	-Dannon -Light 'N Fit Smoothie
1 PM	Lunch	-McDonald's Cheeseburger -Side salad
4 PM	Snack	-Granola Bar (Low-Fat)
7 PM	Dinner	-Healthy Choice Tuna Casserole -Side salad
10 PM	Treat	-Reese's Peanut Butter Cup
↓	⊗ ⊗ ⊗ ⊗ ⊗ ⊗ ⊗ ⊗	

that's great! I highly recommend it. However, most of us don't have time to spend hours making a tomato sauce. Again, I always look to convenience to help me out. But there are countless varieties of prepared foods available, so how do I choose the right ones? Well, I say choose the variety that you like. After all, the 3-Hour Diet™ is about convenience and eating the foods that you love. Maintaining a healthy weight is a lifelong process, so it needs to fit into our daily lives.

Here are some easy guidelines to keep in mind while shopping for prepared items:

- Marinara sauces: Stick to vegetable-based sauces, like tomato basil or mushroom. Meat-based sauces, like Italian sausage, add a lot of additional calories.

- Salad dressings: Each recipe that calls for a prepared salad dressing specifies low-fat or fat free as appropriate to that meal. Stick to vinaigrettes as much as possible, because they have less saturated fat than mayonnaise-based dressings. However, if you like a particular low-fat or nonfat creamy dressing, then use it! Just be sure to stick to the quantity allocated in the recipe.

- Barbecue sauces: Most barbecue sauces are low in fat, but they can be high in sugar, which will increase the calorie load. Look for low-sugar varieties whenever possible.

- Cooked chicken: Many supermarkets carry cooked rotisserie chickens that are perfect for recipes that call for cooked chicken meat. If rotisserie chickens aren't available at your local grocery store, you can probably find packaged chicken breast cuts in the cold-cut section. Whichever you choose, just make sure that you keep your portion size to three ounces.

Fats and Oils

We try to use cooking spray instead of oils whenever possible, but you'll find that a number of the recipes call for olive oil or butter. It's important to have some fat in your diet—it helps you feel more full, it transports fat-soluble vitamins and minerals through your bloodstream, and it makes food taste good—but not too much because it's high in calories. Olive oil is high in heart-healthy monounsaturated fat, so I prefer it to butter, which is high in artery-clogging saturated fat.

Some of the recipes in this book call for extra virgin olive oil and others just list olive oil. What's the difference between the two? Well, extra virgin olive oil comes from the first cold pressing of ripe olives. It's very expensive and full of delicate flavors and aromas that are destroyed by high heat. If you're going to fork over the money for extra virgin (and it *is* worth it) use it when its flavor will really pop and enhance the flavor of the food. A good example of an appropriate use of extra virgin olive oil is the Salmon and Brown Rice recipe. Here, the olive oil is drizzled over steamed veggies. The rich olive flavor enhances the flavor of the veggies and gives body to the side dish.

Other olive oils, such as virgin, pure, and light (which just means light-

BETTER BUTTER

Better Butter is a spreadable, healthier alternative to margarine that has half the saturated fat of butter. It has no partially hydrogenated oils, which research shows are bad for your health. Use Better Butter in place of margarine for your toast or baked potato. See recipes throughout this cookbook for more suggestions on how to use Better Butter.

1 stick (4 ounces) salted butter
¼ teaspoon salt
4 ounces Barlean's® organic flaxseed oil

1. Cut the butter into cubes and gently melt in a small saucepan. Stir in the salt.

2. Pour the liquefied butter into a small, sealable container.

3. Stir in the flaxseed oil. Seal and set in refrigerator to solidify. This will produce a spreadable butter that resembles margarine.

tasting, not lower in fat) are made with the second and third pressings of the olives. They don't have the same fruity flavor as the extra virgin and also don't carry its high price tag. These olive oils are perfect for sautéing, grilling, or roasting. They still have the health benefits of extra virgin olive oil, but you won't waste expensive oil where it won't be appreciated.

So, now you have an overview of what tools and foods will make a reality of losing weight and keeping it off. Remember, incorporating healthy dieting habits into your lifestyle must be simple and convenient in order to be sustainable. Outfitting your kitchen as I outlined above is a first step on the road to free yourself from weight problems.

MARIA BRANDMAIER
LOST 155 POUNDS!

Height: 5' 7"
Age: 40
Starting weight: 310 lbs.
Current weight: 155 lbs.
About Maria: Happily married, stay-at-home mom of three children.

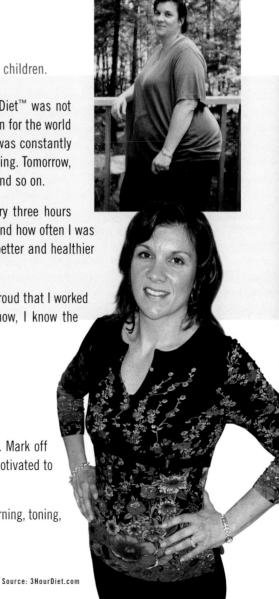

"The image in the mirror before I started Jorge Cruise's 3-Hour Diet™ was not me. I did not know who that person was. I felt I was wearing a sign for the world to see that said 'undisciplined woman who can't lose weight.' I was constantly thinking about my weight. I would tell myself, 'I need to do something. Tomorrow, I will be good. I'll never be able to lose over a hundred pounds,' and so on.

"From the very first day, I knew this was different. Eating every three hours helped me focus on what I was eating, how much I was eating, and how often I was eating. It helped me stop all the 'mindless eating' and to make better and healthier choices.

"I'm now a woman taking charge of her health and her life. I'm proud that I worked hard and sweated off every pound. When I look in the mirror now, I know the woman who is looking back at me."

MARIA'S SECRETS TO SUCCESS

• Make lists. Plan ahead for the next day and just do it!

• Buy a journal to keep track of your eating and exercise routine. Mark off every day that you exercise. Once you see all the marks, you'll be motivated to keep it up.

• Add in Jorge's 8 Minutes in the Morning® exercises for more fat burning, toning, and firming!

Source: 3HourDiet.com

Chapter 3 PICK A QUICK START PLAN

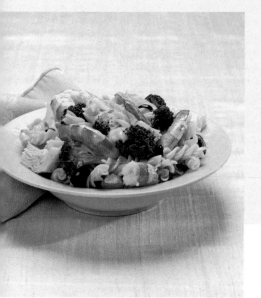

About two years ago, I interviewed more than 300 of my most successful 3HourDiet.com clients. One of the most valuable secrets I learned from them is that those who had a *specific* plan were the most successful. Think about it. If you're going to build a house, you need a blueprint, right? Well, losing weight is no different. You need a plan or a blueprint to clearly show how you're going to construct your new style of eating—and your new style of eating will construct your new, lean, healthy body.

To ensure your success, I've created this optional chapter that offers four different meal plans to allow you to customize the 3-Hour Diet™ to fit your tastes and lifestyle. These four meal plans—Meat Lover, Carb Lover, Healthy Heart, and Veggie—were developed by me and my culinary team. Our goal is to offer you the variety and flexibility you need to be successful in your weight loss efforts. They were further tested and approved by my online clients, who loved the ease with which they could implement them into their busy schedules.

Each meal on the plan is 400 calories. Each snack is 100 calories. And the desserts are 50 calories. Moreover, because each entrée is equal to the other nutritionally, you can swap meals from day to day, menu to menu, or even from meal to meal! You can have the Carb Lover's breakfast for Monday instead of the Meat Lover's dinner on Friday if you want. It can't be simpler.

It may seem hard to believe that losing weight could be this simple and easy. That's why I challenge you to commit to one of these plans. Try it for fourteen days, and get ready to lose up to 10 pounds. If your response is anything like my other clients', you won't believe the benefits that committing to the 3-Hour Diet™ and having a plan for success can make.

Let's take a look at the four different plans you have to choose from:

The Four Quick Start Plans

The four plans below are based on extensive research, polling, discussion, and comments from my 3HourDiet.com clients. Through this research, I discovered that there are four major categories of preferences: Meat Lovers, Carb Lovers, Healthy Heart eaters, and Vegetarians. I therefore crafted the 3-Hour Diet™ Quick Start Plans to accommodate each preference.

Remember that each of these four plans is just as healthy as the other, because they all have the proper balance of protein, carbohydrate, and fat. Therefore, the Meat Lover plan is just as conducive to weight loss as the Veggie plan. That means that you can eat the foods you love and still lose weight!

Meat Lover

When you go out to a restaurant, do you automatically check out the steak and chop section of the menu instead of the pasta? If so, then the Meat Lover meal plan is probably for you. This plan is based primarily on hearty meats: sausage, pork, and cuts of beef. You will be able to choose from Turkey, Bacon, and Egg wrap for breakfast; Hot, Open-Faced Roast Beef Sandwich for lunch; and Filet Mignon with Blue Cheese, Mixed Veggies, and a Baked Potato for dinner. The best part about this plan is that, if you keep to lean cuts of meat, you're able to eat the food you love and maintain your diet effectively.

Carb Lover

Who doesn't love a carb, especially since the low-carb diet trend turned pasta, potatoes, and sugar into forbidden fruit? Well, contrary to the high-protein, low-carb philosophy, you *can* eat carbs and still lose weight. Take a look at our Carb Lover plan, and you will see entrees such as Stuffed Pancakes for breakfast; Potato Stuffed with Broccoli and Melted Cheddar for lunch; and Turkey and Spinach Lasagna for dinner. And, since all of these entrées are only 400 calories, you can indulge in your favorite foods without sabotaging your weight loss efforts.

Healthy Heart

The Healthy Heart plan is similar to the Meat Lover plan, but the Healthy Heart plan focuses primarily on white meats, such as chicken or fish, instead of hearty meats like beef and pork. Delicious options in this plan include Baked Cinnamon Apple with Cottage Cheese and Walnuts for breakfast; Mahi Mahi with Grilled Onion Sandwich for lunch; and Cajun Catfish with Sautéed Greens for dinner.

Veggie

Vegetarian diets are typically considered healthy, but they often don't provide enough protein. Not on the 3-Hour Diet™. Just like the other three plans, the Veggie plan provides the nutrients and balance that are critical to ensuring your weight loss. What could be better than Bubbling Cinnamon Toast for breakfast; Mediterranean Pita for lunch; and Vegetarian Chili for dinner? Eat these delicious foods and know that you're helping your body reach its ideal weight.

Snacks

You'll notice that the snacks are the same from menu to menu. But this is part of the secret to how you will lose up to 10 pounds in 14 days. Unlike any other of my 3-Hour Diet™ books, for fourteen days you will be only eating these carefully chosen snacks that are ample in fiber (see page 38).

What Are the Rules of the Quick Start Plans?

So, how do you get started with the Quick Start Plans? Since these plans were designed to be simple and easy, there are only two rules that you need to remember.

Pick a Plan

Yes, the first rule really is that easy. Are you a Meat Lover? A Carb Lover? Or do you prefer vegetarian meals? It's entirely up to you. You choose your plan solely on which foods you like to eat.

Stick to the Plan

When following these plans you need to only eat what is offered and eat every three hours. That means that you must stick to the caloric limits—400-calorie meals, 100-calorie snacks, and a 50-calorie treat—and not overindulge. Overeating will sabotage your efforts. Remember, it's important to eat every three hours to keep your blood sugar steady and stave off the starvation protection mechanism.

Fourteen days is all you need to commit to in order for you too see the results of your hard work. In fourteen days, up to 10 pounds of fat will have melted off your body. The fiber you have been eating will have flushed out your digestive system, eliminating false fat and that bulge in your tummy. Your appetite will be under control, and you will feel more energized. Choose a meal plan and embark on the most important two weeks of your life.

Take a look at the delicious meals suggested in the following plans and choose one that best suits your lifestyle.

MEAT LOVER

	1	2	3	4	5	6	7
Breakfast	Egg White and Sausage Sandwich (page 53)	Breakfast Ham and Cheese (page 78)	Breakfast Sausage Biscuits (page 65)	Ham and Ricotta Pita (page 66)	Turkey, Bacon, and Egg Wrap (page 55)	Oats with Turkey Bacon (page 75)	Egg White and Sausage Sandwich (page 53)
Snack	Cheesy Popcorn (page 291)	10 Orville Redenbacher's® Popcorn Mini Cakes, all flavors (page 309)	1 Nature Valley® Granola Bar, all flavors (page 308)	1 banana (page 308)	3 prunes/ dried plums (page 308)	Three-Bean Salad (page 294)	Taco Broccoli (page 304)
Lunch	Roast Beef and Swiss Cheese Sandwich (page 218)	Roast Beef and Provolone Wraps (page 223)	Hot Open-Faced Roast Beef Sandwich (page 231)	Cheese-burger Pie with Mixed Greens (page 194)	Honey Mustard Ham Pita (page 246)	Pork Chops with Squash Soup (page 203)	Sliced Pizza Burger (page 226)
Snack	Cereal Trail Mix (page 291)	Veggies and Dip (page 301)	12 almonds (page 309)	1 medium apple, green or red (page 308)	30 raisins (page 308)	24 grapes, green or red (page 308)	Pita with Hummus (page 301)
Dinner	Meatloaf Patties (page 186)	Marinated Flank Steak (page 185)	Pork-and-Pineapple Kebabs with Mixed Greens (page 204)	Pork Chops with Squash Soup (page 203)	Filet Mignon Topped with Blue Cheese, Mixed Veggies, and a Baked Potato (page 191)	Grilled Blackened Skirt Steak (page 187)	Blackened Pork Chops with Yams and Steamed Broccoli (page 207)
Dessert	Chocolate-Covered Strawberries (page 313)	1 cup frozen seedless grapes	Frozen Banana Ice Cream (page 319)	Cinnamon Sugar Popcorn (page 326)	Yogurt Parfait (page 326)	Strawberry Shortcake (page 316)	Ladyfinger Parfait (page 314)

8	9	10	11	12	13	14
Turkey, Bacon, and Egg Wrap (page 55)	Breakfast Sausage Biscuits (page 65)	Ham and Ricotta Pita (page 66)	Breakfast Ham and Cheese (page 78)	Oats with Turkey Bacon (page 75)	Ham and Ricotta Pita (page 66)	Breakfast Ham and Cheese (page 78)
Cheesy Popcorn (page 291)	10 Orville Reden-bacher's® Popcorn Mini Cakes, all flavors (page 309)	1 Nature Valley® Granola Bar, all flavors (page 308)	1 banana (page 308)	3 prunes/dried plums (page 308)	Three-Bean Salad (page 294)	Taco Broccoli (page 304)
Honey Mustard Ham Pita (page 246)	Roast Beef and Swiss Cheese Sandwich (page 218)	Roast Beef and Provolone Wraps (page 223)	Hot Open-Faced Roast Beef Sandwich (page 231)	Honey Mustard Ham Pita (page 246)	Cheeseburger Pie with Mixed Greens (page 194)	Sliced Pizza Burger (page 226)
Cereal Trail Mix (page 291)	Veggies and Dip (page 301)	12 almonds (page 309)	1 medium apple, green or red (page 308)	30 raisins (page 308)	24 grapes, green or red (page 308)	Pita with Hummus (page 301)
Grilled Pork with Mango Salsa over Rice, and Carrots (page 210)	Pork Teriyaki with Couscous (page 209)	Apricot Pork over Rice with Mixed Veggies (page 212)	Grilled Pork Cutlets with Citrus Salsa (page 200)	Barbecued Flank Steak with Grilled Veggies and Rice (page 192)	Grilled Sirloin Steak with Mustard Sauce, Rice and Broccoli (page 196)	Grilled Sirloin Patties with Onion-Mushroom Sauce and Couscous (page 198)
Chocolate-Covered Strawberries (page 313)	1 cup frozen seedless grapes	Frozen Banana Ice Cream (page 319)	Cinnamon Sugar Popcorn (page 326)	Yogurt Parfait (page 326)	Strawberry Shortcake (page 316)	Ladyfinger Parfait (page 314)

CARB LOVER

	1	2	3	4	5	6	7
Breakfast	Breakfast Banana Split (page 76)	Cereal with Milk and Cottage Cheese (page 84)	Stuffed Pancakes (page 73)	Egg Breakfast Burrito (page 57)	Breakfast Smoothie (page 96)	Ricotta Cheese Toast (page 70)	Egg Sandwich (page 52)
Snack	Cheesy Popcorn (page 291)	10 Orville Redenbacher's® Popcorn Mini Cakes, all flavors (page 309)	1 Nature Valley® Granola Bar, all flavors (page 308)	1 banana (page 308)	3 prunes/ dried plums (page 308)	Three-Bean Salad (page 294)	Taco Broccoli (page 304)
Lunch	Three-Cheese Pizza (page 123)	Barbecued Turkey Burger (page 238)	Pizza Tapenade with Mozzarella (page 125)	Taco Salad (page 251)	Potato Stuffed with Broccoli and Melted Cheddar (page 276)	Honey Mustard Ham Pita (page 246)	Sliced Pizza Burger (page 226)
Snack	Cereal Trail Mix (page 291)	Veggies and Dip (page 301)	12 almonds (page 309)	1 medium apple, green or red (page 308)	30 raisins (page 308)	24 grapes, green or red (page 308)	Pita with Hummus (page 301)
Dinner	Turkey and Spinach Lasagna (page 108)	Pineapple Ricotta Pizza (page 122)	Gnocchi with Turkey Sausage and Spinach (page 112)	Pizza Tapenade with Mozzarella (page 125)	Fusilli Pasta with Shrimp and Artichokes (page 102)	Grilled Chicken, Artichoke, and Goat Cheese Pizza (page 116)	Turkey Sausage Pasta with Kale (page 101)
Dessert	Chocolate-Covered Strawberries (page 313)	1 cup frozen seedless grapes	Frozen Banana Ice Cream (page 319)	Cinnamon Sugar Popcorn (page 326)	Yogurt Parfait (page 326)	Strawberry Shortcake (page 316)	Ladyfinger Parfait (page 314)

8	9	10	11	12	13	14
Oats with Turkey Bacon (page 75)	Waffle with Cottage Cheese and Fruit (page 74)	Bubbling Cinnamon Toast (page 68)	Waffles with Almond Butter (page 83)	Cereal with Milk and Cottage Cheese (page 84)	Fruity Pizza (page 72)	Layered Yogurt Parfait (page 91)
Cheesy Popcorn (page 291)	10 Orville Reden-bacher's® Popcorn Mini Cakes, all flavors (page 309)	1 Nature Valley® Granola Bar, all flavors (page 308)	1 banana (page 308)	3 prunes/dried plums (page 308)	Three-Bean Salad (page 294)	Taco Broccoli (page 304)
Roast Beef and Swiss Cheese Sandwich (page 218)	Chili and Potatoes (page 168)	Chicken Waldorf Salad (page 261)	Turkey Tortilla Wrap (page 239)	Mozzarella Cheese Melt (page 227)	Open-Faced Tuna Veggie Melts (page 228)	Grilled Shrimp Caesar Salad (page 262)
Cereal Trail Mix (page 291)	Veggies and Dip (page 301)	12 almonds (page 309)	1 medium apple, green or red (page 308)	30 raisins (page 308)	24 grapes, green or red (page 308)	Pita with Hummus (page 301)
Three-Cheese Pizza (page 123)	Penne Pasta with Chicken and Mixed Veggies (page 105)	Fresh Tomato and Mozzarella Pizza (page 119)	Spaghetti with Meat Sauce and Caesar Salad (page 111)	Blue Cheese, Red Onion, and Olive Pizza (page 120)	Tomato Sauce over Linguini with Tuna and Capers (page 106)	White Pizza with Basil (page 124)
Chocolate-Covered Strawberries (page 313)	1 cup frozen seedless grapes	Frozen Banana Ice Cream (page 319)	Cinnamon Sugar Popcorn (page 326)	Yogurt Parfait (page 326)	Strawberry Shortcake (page 316)	Ladyfinger Parfait (page 314)

HEALTHY HEART

	1	2	3	4	5	6	7
Breakfast	Cottage Cheese with Granola and Fresh Fruit (page 84)	Fruity Pizza (page 72)	Poached Delight (page 45)	Layered Yogurt Parfait (page 91)	Egg Breakfast Burrito (page 57)	Baked Cinnamon Apple with Cottage Cheese and Walnuts (page 77)	Scrambled Eggs with English Muffins (page 58)
Snack	Cheesy Popcorn (page 291)	10 Orville Redenbacher's® Popcorn Mini Cakes, all flavors (page 309)	1 Nature Valley® Granola Bar, all flavors (page 308)	1 banana (page 308)	3 prunes/ dried plums (page 308)	Three-Bean Salad (page 294)	Taco Broccoli (page 304)
Lunch	Tuna, Bean, and Vegetable Salad (page 255)	Turkey Sandwich and Coleslaw (page 220)	Salmon Salad (page 258)	Chunky Turkey Salad with Cranberries and Walnuts (page 265)	Salmon Burgers and Sugar Snap Peas (page 242)	Mahimahi with Sweet Onion Sandwich (page 236)	Smoked Turkey and Mozzarella Wrap (page 220)
Snack	Cereal Trail Mix (page 291)	Veggies and Dip (page 301)	12 almonds (page 309)	1 medium apple, green or red (page 308)	30 raisins (page 308)	24 grapes, green or red (page 308)	Pita with Hummus (page 301)
Dinner	Spaghetti with Meat Sauce and Caesar Salad (page 111)	Tomato Sauce over Linguini with Tuna and Capers (page 106)	Quick Fish Tacos (page 140)	Grilled Chicken with Mango Corn Salsa (page 165)	Grilled Italian Chicken (page 174)	Chili and Potatoes (page 168)	Cajun Catfish with Sautéed Greens (page 154)
Dessert	Chocolate-Covered Strawberries (page 313)	1 cup frozen seedless grapes	Frozen Banana Ice Cream (page 319)	Cinnamon Sugar Popcorn (page 326)	Yogurt Parfait (page 326)	Strawberry Shortcake (page 316)	Ladyfinger Parfait (page 314)

8	9	10	11	12	13	14
Vanilla Yogurt and Berry Parfait (page 88)	Waffle with Cottage Cheese and Fruit (page 74)	Apples, Walnuts, and Yogurt (page 92)	Bubbling Cinnamon Toast (page 68)	Strawberry-Banana Yogurt Shake (page 95)	Vegetable Frittata (page 49)	Breakfast Smoothie (page 96)
Cheesy Popcorn (page 291)	10 Orville Reden-bacher's® Popcorn Mini Cakes, all flavors (page 309)	1 Nature Valley® Granola Bar, all flavors (page 308)	1 banana (page 308)	3 prunes/dried plums (page 308)	Three-Bean Salad (page 294)	Taco Broccoli (page 304)
Cold Tuna Platter (page 131)	Smoked Turkey and Mozzarella Wrap (page 220)	Salmon Burgers and Sugar Snap Peas (page 242)	Turkey and Cranberry Sandwich (page 245)	Quick Chicken Curry with Couscous and Spinach Salad (page 173)	Grilled Shrimp, Hummus, and Veggie Platter (page 132)	Grilled Chicken Gorgonzola Wrap (page 217)
Cereal Trail Mix (page 291)	Veggies and Dip (page 301)	12 almonds (page 309)	1 medium apple, green or red (page 308)	30 raisins (page 308)	24 grapes, green or red (page 308)	Pita with Hummus (page 301)
Chicken and Cheese Tostadas (page 163)	Chili Lime Shrimp with Brown Rice and Toasted Pecans (page 156)	Chicken Burrito with Salsa (page 166)	Sautéed Scallops with Spinach over Polenta (page 146)	Turkey and Spinach Lasagna (page 108)	Turkey Cutlets with Lime Sauce (page 170)	Chili Lime Shrimp with Brown Rice and Toasted Pecans (page 156)
Chocolate-Covered Strawberries (page 313)	1 cup frozen seedless grapes	Frozen Banana Ice Cream (page 319)	Cinnamon Sugar Popcorn (page 326)	Yogurt Parfait (page 326)	Strawberry Shortcake (page 316)	Ladyfinger Parfait (page 314)

VEGGIE

	1	2	3	4	5	6	7
Breakfast	Fruity Pizza (page 72)	Layered Yogurt Parfait (page 91)	Peanut Butter and Banana (page 81)	Soy Cranberry Shake with Peanut Butter Toast (page 89)	Bubbling Cinnamon Toast (page 68)	Vanilla Yogurt and Berry Parfait (page 88)	Veggie Sausage and Egg Sandwich (page 56)
Snack	Cheesy Popcorn (page 291)	10 Orville Reden-bacher's® Popcorn Mini Cakes, all flavors (page 309)	1 Nature Valley® Granola Bar, all flavors (page 308)	1 banana (page 308)	3 prunes/ dried plums (page 308)	Three-Bean Salad (page 294)	Taco Broccoli (page 304)
Lunch	Chickpea Vegetable Curry (page 279)	Mediterra-nean Pita (page 284)	Miso Soup with Soba Noodles (page 283)	Spinach Salad (page 267)	Spinach Beet Salad (page 256)	Grilled Hawaiian Soy Burger (page 281)	Pineapple Ricotta Pizza (page 122)
Snack	Cereal Trail Mix (page 291)	Veggies and Dip (page 301)	12 almonds (page 309)	1 medium apple, green or red (page 308)	30 raisins (page 308)	24 grapes, green or red (page 308)	Pita with Hummus (page 301)
Dinner	Grilled Eggplant Parmesan (page 271)	Vegetarian Chili (page 272)	Potato Stuffed with Broccoli and Melted Cheddar (page 276)	Burrito and Greens (page 274)	Soy Crumble Pitas (page 282)	Franks and Beans (page 280)	Garden-burgers® with Vegetable Crudités (page 273)
Dessert	Chocolate-Covered Strawberries (page 313)	1 cup frozen seedless grapes	Frozen Banana Ice Cream (page 319)	Cinnamon Sugar Popcorn (page 326)	Yogurt Parfait (page 326)	Strawberry Shortcake (page 316)	Ladyfinger Parfait (page 314)

8	9	10	11	12	13	14
Breakfast Tacos (page 61)	Apples, Walnuts, and Yogurt (page 92)	Ricotta Cheese Toast (page 70)	Orange and Banana Smoothie (page 96)	Cottage Cheese with Granola and Fresh Fruit (page 84)	Fruity Pizza (page 72)	Breakfast Smoothie (page 96)
Cheesy Popcorn (page 291)	10 Orville Reden-bacher's® Popcorn Mini Cakes, all fla-vors (page 309)	1 Nature Valley® Granola Bar, all flavors (page 308)	1 banana (page 308)	3 prunes/dried plums (page 308)	Three-Bean Salad (page 294)	Taco Broccoli (page 304)
Blue Cheese, Red Onion, and Olive Pizza (page 120)	Potato Stuffed with Broccoli and Melted Cheddar (page 276)	Soy Crumble Pitas (page 282)	Garden Burgers with Vegetable Crudités (page 273)	Mediterranean Pita (Page 284)	Bean Burrito (page 275)	Miso Soup with Soba Noodles (page 283)
Cereal Trail Mix (page 291)	Veggies and Dip (page 301)	12 almonds (page 309)	1 medium apple, green or red (page 308)	30 raisins (page 308)	24 grapes, green or red (page 308)	Pita with Hummus (page 301)
Grilled Hawaiian Soy Burger (page 281)	Bean Burrito (page 275)	Chickpea Vegetable Curry (page 279)	Grilled Eggplant Parmesan (page 271)	Vegetarian Chili (page 272)	Burrito and Greens (page 274)	Tortilla Pizza (page 115)
Chocolate-Covered Strawberries (page 313)	1 cup frozen seedless grapes	Frozen Banana Ice Cream (page 319)	Cinnamon Sugar Popcorn (page 326)	Yogurt Parfait (page 326)	Strawberry Shortcake (page 316)	Ladyfinger Parfait (page 314)

HOW TO AVOID EMOTIONAL EATING

What is emotional eating? It's eating anytime you aren't hungry! It's the number one saboteur of dieters, yet it's often overlooked in most weight loss plans. Well, not this one.

So, how do you overcome this common pitfall? It's called the People Solution™ Plan. Here's how it works. The next time you reach for food when you're not hungry, ask yourself why you're eating. Is that food what you really need? Odds are, the answer is no. So, how do you cope with moments of insecurity, boredom, sadness, or stress without reaching for food? You need to create a safety net of two factors:

1. You need to become your own best friend—fast. You need to *nurture yourself* in this time of need. How do you nurture yourself effectively and quickly? The solution is simple: you need to see your desired future *now*. You need to see the ideal you. Visualize yourself walking tall and confidently. See yourself in control and being decisive with yourself, friends, and family about your meal and food decisions. Envision how happy you are with the slim, sexy body you will work so hard to achieve. Positive visualizations are essential to your success if you are an emotional eater.

2. Create a network of support. This network can include family members, coworkers, and good friends—anyone with whom you feel comfortable communicating with openly and honestly. People in your network of support must be caring and nonjudgmental. They must be willing to genuinely listen to you and support you. Another way to add new people to your network is by connecting online. If you join 3HourDiet.com you will have access to our amazing community of members as well as myself. You and I would be able to connect through a daily video coaching session designed to keep you motivated and focused. Each day, I will share my latest secrets to staying on track and motivated as well as success stories from other 3HourDiet.com clients.

BANISH FALSE FAT!

Eating a lot of fiber is crucial to successful weight loss. Why is fiber important? Well, have you ever noticed a bulge in your abdomen, even after exercising and eating right? That bulge may be the result of what I call "false fat." False fat is the air, fluid, or waste trapped in your belly. Your intestines are a whopping 25 feet long, and when they fail to move digested food efficiently, things get blocked up. The result: your intestines swell and your tummy expands. However, there is a simple cure: eat plenty of fiber to stay regular. That's why our 3-Hour Diet™ offers you so many fiber-rich snacks; not only are they filling, but they also keep you from being weighed down by false fats.

Part 2
MAIN COURSES

Chapter 4
BREAKFAST

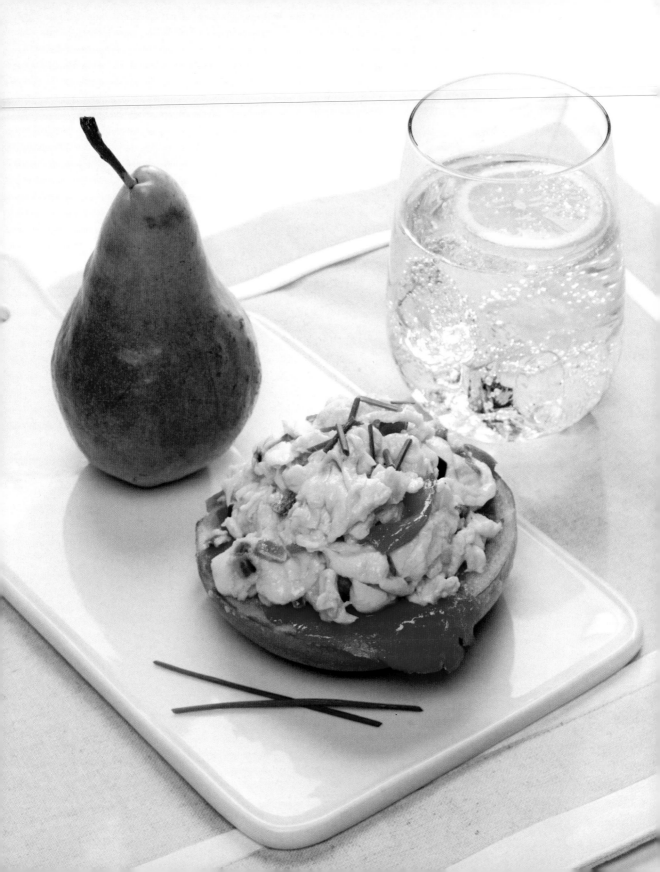

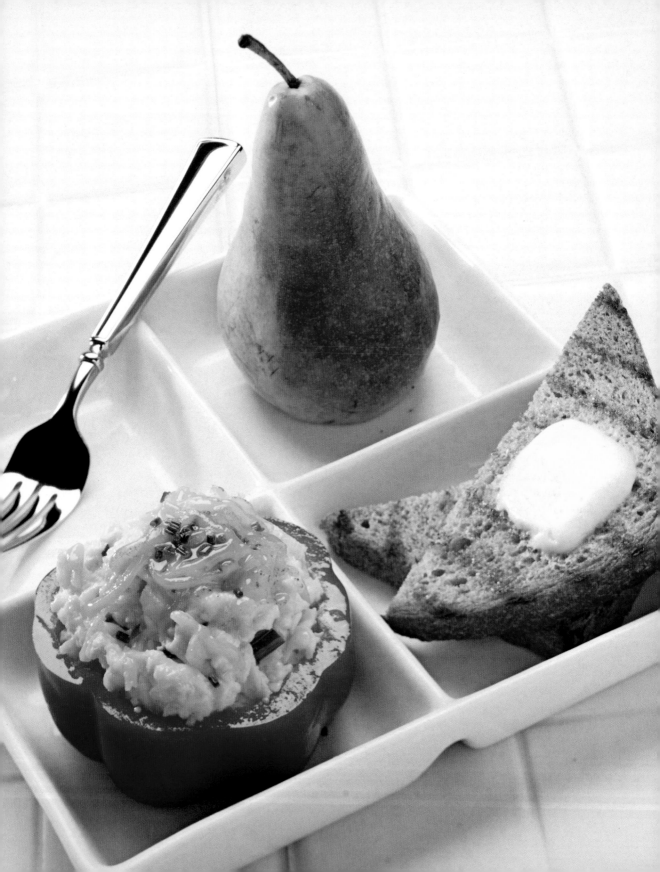

SUPER SCRAMBLED STUFFED PEPPER

Sneak in a morning vegetable with these egg-stuffed bell peppers. The colorful bowl will make this meal an attractive and tasty breakfast.

MAKES 4 SERVINGS

4 red bell peppers, tops and seeds removed
Cooking spray
2 green onions, sliced
8 large eggs, lightly beaten
4 ounces shredded low-fat cheddar, about ½ cup
4 slices whole grain bread
4 teaspoons butter or Better Butter (see page 23)
4 medium pears

1. Preheat the broiler.

2. Microwave the peppers for 2 to 3 minutes to soften. Place the peppers in an oven-safe baking dish and set aside.

3. Spray a nonstick skillet with cooking spray, heat over medium heat, and sauté the onions until soft, 2 minutes.

4. Add the eggs to the onions and scramble until soft curds form, 3 to 4 minutes.

5. Place the egg mixture inside the peppers and top with the cheddar.

6. Broil the egg-stuffed peppers until the cheese is melted, 1 minute.

7. Toast and butter the bread while the peppers broil.

8. Serve each person one stuffed pepper, one slice of buttered toast, and one pear.

TURKEY BREAKFAST WRAP

Egg whites provide the highest quality protein you can find. However, egg substitutes approximate whole eggs better when scrambled, so give a product like Egg Beaters® a try and see if you like it. Egg substitutes are made primarily of egg whites, with flavoring and thickening agents, and have no cholesterol.

MAKES 4 SERVINGS

Four 1-ounce slices smoked turkey breast
Cooking spray
12 large egg whites or equivalent egg substitute
Four 6-inch flour tortillas
Four 1-ounce slices Swiss cheese
4 medium apples

1. Heat a nonstick skillet over medium heat.

2. Dice the turkey into 2-inch pieces and add to the skillet. Cook until the turkey starts to brown, 2 minutes. Remove the turkey from the pan and set aside.

3. Spray the skillet with cooking spray and place again over medium heat.

4. Lightly beat the egg whites in a small bowl. Add the egg whites to the skillet and cook until they start to form curds, about 2 to 3 minutes. Return the turkey to the pan and cook until the eggs are set, 3 to 4 minutes.

5. Divide the eggs among the four tortillas, top with the cheese, and roll into burrito shapes.

6. Serve each person one tortilla wrap with one apple.

POACHED DELIGHT

This fulfilling meal is perfect for a relaxing Sunday morning brunch. To keep your egg white from spreading out, add just a drizzle or two of white vinegar to the water before poaching the egg.

MAKES 4 SERVINGS

2 whole grain English muffins, halved
4 teaspoons butter or Better Butter (see page 23)
Four 2-ounce slices Canadian bacon
4 slices 2% American cheese
4 slices tomato
4 large eggs
4 medium peaches

1. Bring 2 inches of water to a simmer over medium heat in a large sauté pan.

2. Toast and butter the English muffins.

3. Place one piece of Canadian bacon on each English muffin half and top each one with a slice of cheese. Microwave English muffins for 30 seconds to melt the cheese. Top each with a tomato slice.

4. When the water comes to a simmer, carefully slip in the eggs. Poach eggs (do not boil) until whites set, 3 to 4 minutes. Carefully remove the poached eggs with a slotted spoon and dry on paper towels.

5. Place one egg on top of each English muffin half.

6. Serve each person one English muffin half with one peach.

LOX AND EGG BAGEL

Lox, salmon fillet that has been cured and then sometimes smoked, is often served with bagels. Our recipe adds eggs and sautéed onions for a special breakfast indulgence.

MAKES 4 SERVINGS

Two 2-ounce frozen bagels, halved
4 teaspoons butter or Better Butter (see page 23)
Cooking spray
1 cup chopped onions (tip: buy pre-chopped, frozen onions)
4 ounces lox, diced
4 large eggs, lightly beaten
12 large egg whites, lightly beaten
1 tablespoon chopped fresh chives
4 medium pears

1. Toast the bagels and spread with butter. Place on four plates.

2. Heat a large nonstick skillet over medium heat and spray with cooking spray.

3. Add the onions to the pan and sauté until translucent, 4 minutes.

4. Add the lox and sauté until warmed through, 2 minutes.

5. Add the eggs and egg whites and scramble until cooked through, 4 minutes.

6. Top each bagel with one-fourth of the egg mixture and garnish with chives.

7. Serve each person one bagel half with one pear.

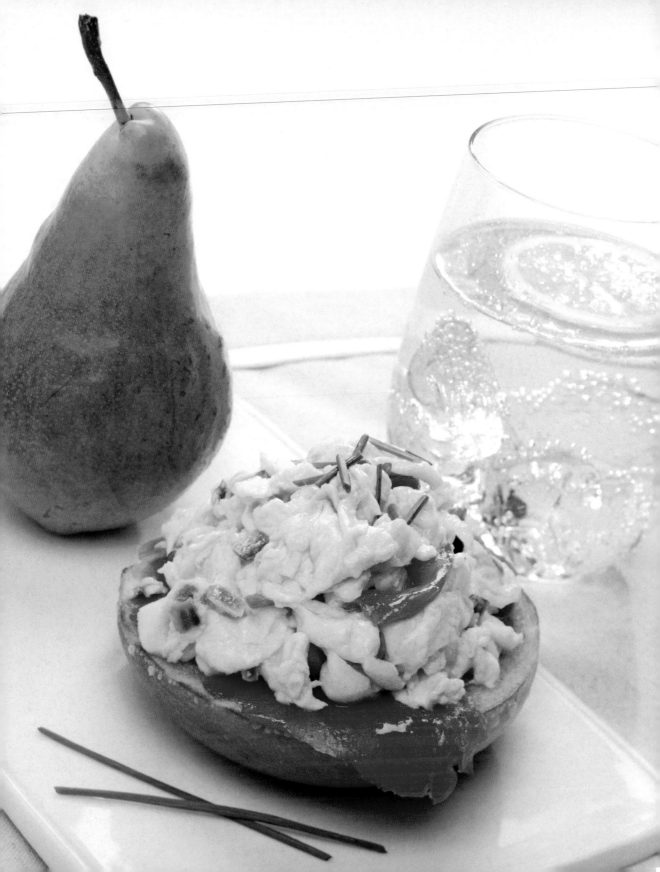

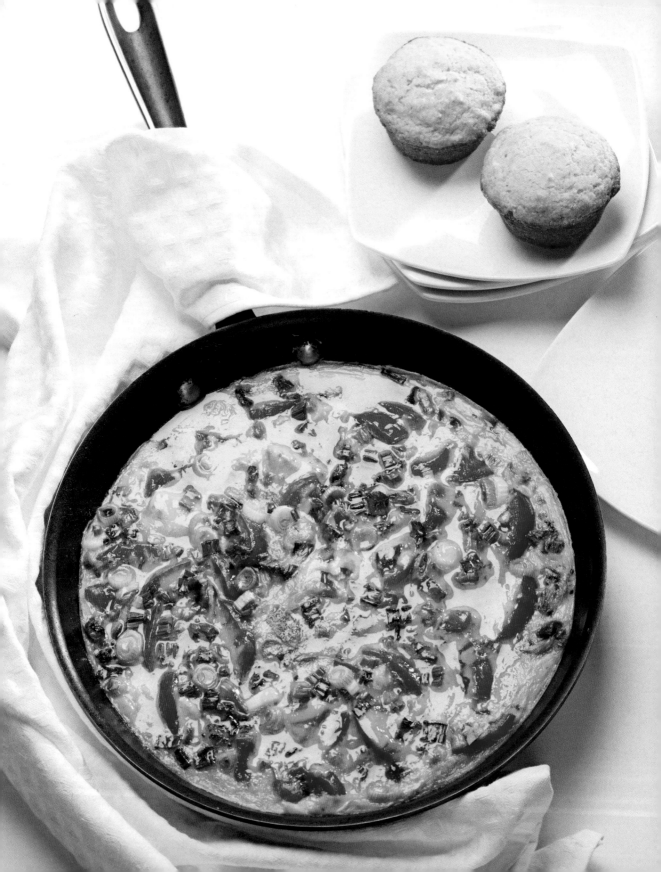

VEGETABLE FRITTATA

A frittata is a type of Italian omelet that can have a variety of fillings, such as the mixed vegetables in this one. Use frozen, chopped vegetables to prepare this breakfast in no time.

MAKES 4 SERVINGS

Cooking spray
1 tablespoon olive oil
1 cup diced onion
1 cup diced bell peppers
1 cup sliced mushrooms
1 cup chopped broccoli
8 large eggs, lightly beaten
1 tomato, diced
2 green onions, chopped
4 ounces shredded low-fat cheddar, about ½ cup
4 small corn muffins

1. Preheat the broiler.

2. Heat a heavy, oven-proof nonstick skillet over medium-high heat. Spray with cooking spray and add the olive oil.

3. Add the onion, peppers, mushrooms, and broccoli and cook until softened, 2 to 3 minutes. Add the eggs, stir to combine, and cook until mostly set, 3 to 4 minutes.

4. Top with the tomato, green onions, and cheese. Place the pan under the broiler until the cheese is melted and the top is set, 2 minutes.

5. Cut the frittata into four pieces and serve each person one slice with one muffin.

BREAKFAST STUFFED PEPPERS

Made with mild poblano chile peppers or Anaheim peppers, this fabulous meal is perfect to serve when you have company or as a special family breakfast.

MAKES 4 SERVINGS

4 green poblano or Anaheim peppers
Cooking spray
1 cup chopped tomatoes, about 4 medium
4 large eggs, lightly beaten
8 large egg whites, lightly beaten
4 ounces shredded low-fat Swiss cheese, about ½ cup
4 teaspoons butter
4 slices white bread, diced into small cubes

1. Preheat broiler.

2. Slice the peppers in half lengthwise. Remove the seeds and broil until the peppers soften, 3 to 4 minutes. Drain any water that surfaces and set aside.

3. While the peppers broil, heat a large nonstick skillet over medium heat and spray with cooking spray.

4. Add the tomatoes to skillet and sauté until softened, 1 minute. Add eggs and whites to the tomatoes and scramble untii nearly set, 3 to 4 minutes. Stir in the cheese until melted. Remove from heat.

5. Heat another skillet over medium-high heat and add the butter while the eggs cook. When the butter is melted, add the bread cubes and cook until browned.

6. Add the bread cubes to egg mixture and fold in gently.

7. Stuff each pepper half with one-eighth of the bread and egg mixture.

8. Serve each person two pepper halves.

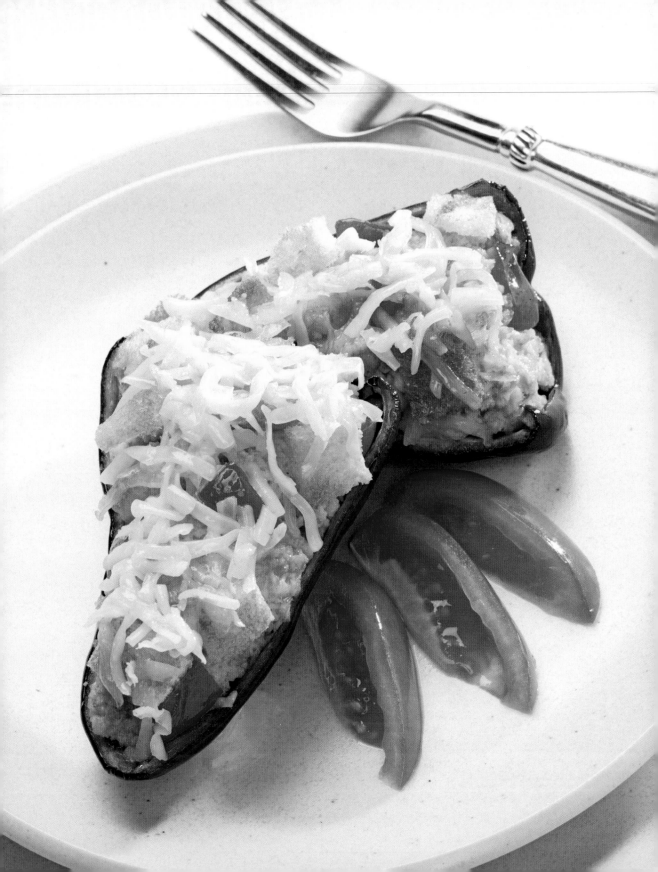

EGG SANDWICH

Spinach not only tastes great, it's also a rich source of iron, calcium, vitamin A, vitamin C, vitamin E, and several vital antioxidants. If you prefer, you can replace the spinach with any other dark green, such as chard, mustard greens, or collard greens. To make this meal super convenient, look for prewashed, bagged baby greens at the supermarket.

MAKES 4 SERVINGS

Cooking spray
8 slices turkey bacon, chopped
4 large eggs, lightly beaten
4 large egg whites, lightly beaten
2 cups baby spinach
4 ounces shredded cheddar, about ½ cup
8 slices whole grain bread
4 tablespoons stone-ground mustard

1. Heat a nonstick skillet over medium heat and spray with cooking spray.

2. Add the bacon pieces and sauté until crisp, 4 minutes.

3. Add the eggs, egg whites, spinach, and cheese. Cook until the bottom is set, 3 to 4 minutes. Periodically lift the cooked edges with a spatula and tilt pan to allow uncooked egg to run underneath.

4. Toast the bread while the eggs are cooking.

5. When the bottom of the omelet is cooked and the top is nearly set, fold one-third of the omelet over itself with a spatula. Slide the folded edge onto a plate and, using the pan to help you, fold the opposite side of the omelet over, creating a trifold.

6. Slice omelet into fourths and place one piece on each slice of toast. Top with mustard and remaining four slices of toast.

EGG WHITE AND SAUSAGE SANDWICH

For those who are looking to enjoy a meatless breakfast, this open-faced sandwich with a soy crumble–egg white topping is a delicious alternative. Also known as textured vegetable protein, soy crumbles can be used as a meat substitute in any recipe that calls for ground beef, chicken, or turkey.

MAKES 4 SERVINGS

4 teaspoons olive oil
8 ounces sausage-style soy crumbles
12 large egg whites, lightly beaten
4 slices whole grain bread
4 slices 2% American cheese
4 slices honeydew melon (⅛ melon each)

1.   Heat a large nonstick skillet over medium-high heat and add the olive oil.

2.   Add the soy crumbles and brown, breaking them up as you cook.

3.   Add the egg whites and scramble until soft curds form, 3 to 4 minutes.

4.   Toast the bread while the eggs cook. Place one piece of toast on each of four plates.

5.   Place one-fourth of the sausage-egg mixture on each piece of toast and top with cheese, which should melt from the heat of the egg mixture.

6.   Serve each person one open-faced sandwich with one slice of melon.

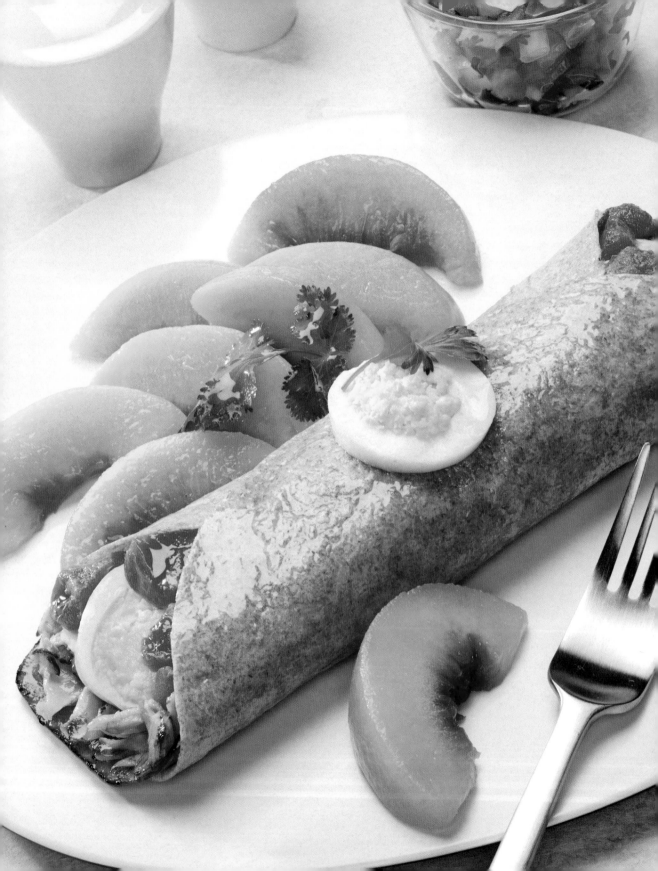

TURKEY, BACON, AND EGG WRAP

Wraps are simple, quick, and easy to make. You'll only need one pan and a few minutes to create this mouthwatering turkey-and-bacon wrap.

MAKES 4 SERVINGS

4 teaspoons olive oil
1 cup chopped tomatoes, about 4 medium
Four 1-ounce slices turkey breast
Four 1-ounce slices Canadian bacon
4 hard-boiled eggs, sliced
Four 6-inch flour tortillas
4 small peaches

1. Heat a large nonstick skillet over medium-high heat and add the olive oil.

2. Add the tomatoes and sauté until soft, 1 minute. Put the tomatoes on a plate and return the skillet to heat.

3. Add turkey and bacon to the skillet and cook until lightly browned, 3 to 4 minutes.

4. Add one slice of turkey, one slice of Canadian bacon, and one sliced egg to each tortilla. Top with the tomatoes and roll into a burrito shape.

5. Serve each person one wrap with one peach.

VEGGIE SAUSAGE AND EGG SANDWICH

Serve these fantastic veggie sausages and eggs between two halves of a whole grain English muffin. Whole grains retain the bran and germ of the grain and therefore provide more fiber and nutrients than refined grains.

MAKES 4 SERVINGS

4 Morningstar Farms® vegetarian sausage patties
Cooking spray
4 large eggs, lightly beaten
4 whole grain English muffins, halved
4 tablespoons mustard
3 cups strawberries or fruit in season (thawed if frozen)

1. Heat two nonstick skillets over medium heat.

2. Add the veggie patties to one skillet and sauté until they brown and crisp, 5 minutes per side.

3. Spray the other skillet with cooking spray. Add the eggs and scramble until they set, 3 to 4 minutes.

4. Toast the English muffins while the sausage and eggs cook.

5. Spread the bottom half of each muffin with mustard. Top with one sausage patty and one-fourth of the eggs, then add the top half of the muffin.

6. Serve each person one sandwich with ¾ cup of fruit.

EGG BREAKFAST BURRITO

A flavorful variation on traditional scrambled eggs and toast, this recipe calls for whole eggs and egg whites, which reduces the fat but increases the lean protein in this dish.

MAKES 4 SERVINGS

Four 6-inch whole wheat tortillas
½ teaspoon olive oil
2 large eggs
4 large egg whites
Salt and freshly ground black pepper
4 ounces shredded cheese (cheddar or pepper Jack would work well), about ½ cup
1 cup prepared salsa
4 medium apples

1. Heat tortillas in a microwave for 1 minute. Wrap in foil to keep warm.

2. Meanwhile, heat a large nonstick skillet over medium-high heat and add the olive oil.

3. Whisk the eggs, egg whites, 2 tablespoons water, and a pinch of salt and freshly ground black pepper to taste in a large bowl.

4. Add the egg mixture to the skillet and cook, stirring often, until the eggs are set, 3 to 4 minutes.

5. Place the tortillas on four plates and divide the scrambled eggs equally among them.

6. Top with the cheese and salsa and roll into a burrito shape.

7. Serve each person one burrito and one apple.

SCRAMBLED EGGS WITH ENGLISH MUFFINS

If you are an egg lover, try this meal. Egg whites provide excellent low-fat protein, and the spinach provides antioxidants, fiber, and tons of vitamin A. This meal is great for breakfast, lunch, and dinner.

MAKES 4 SERVINGS

Cooking spray
1 onion, chopped
4 cups baby spinach
4 large eggs, lightly beaten
8 large egg whites, lightly beaten
¼ cup grated Parmesan
2 whole grain English muffins, halved
2 oranges

1. Heat a large nonstick skillet over medium heat and spray with cooking spray.

2. Add the onion to the skillet and sauté until translucent, 1 to 2 minutes.

3. Add the spinach and cook until wilted, 1 to 2 minutes.

4. Add eggs, egg whites, and Parmesan. Scramble until set, 3 to 4 minutes.

5. Toast the English muffins while the eggs are cooking.

6. Serve each person one-fourth of the scrambled eggs, one English muffin half, and half an orange.

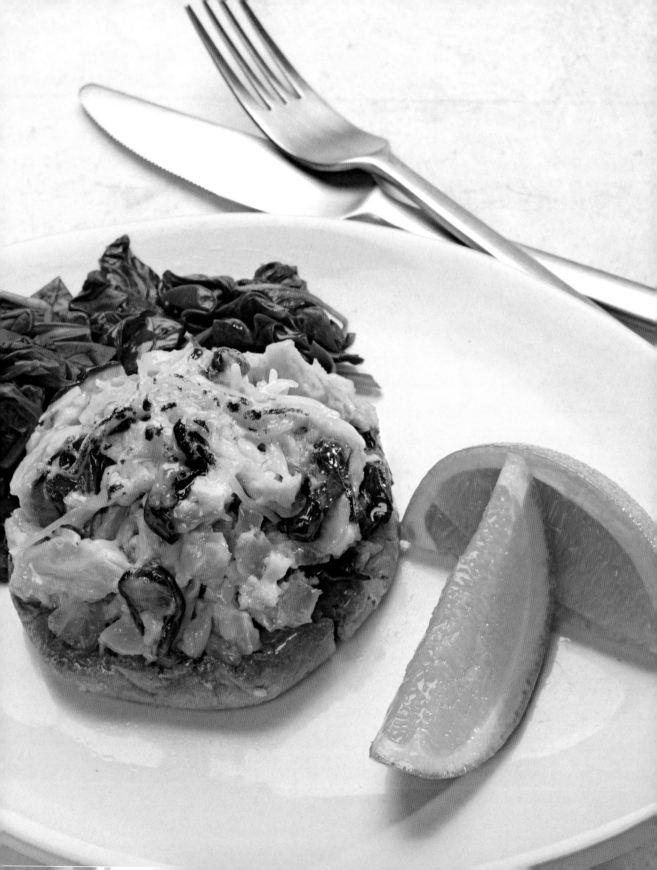

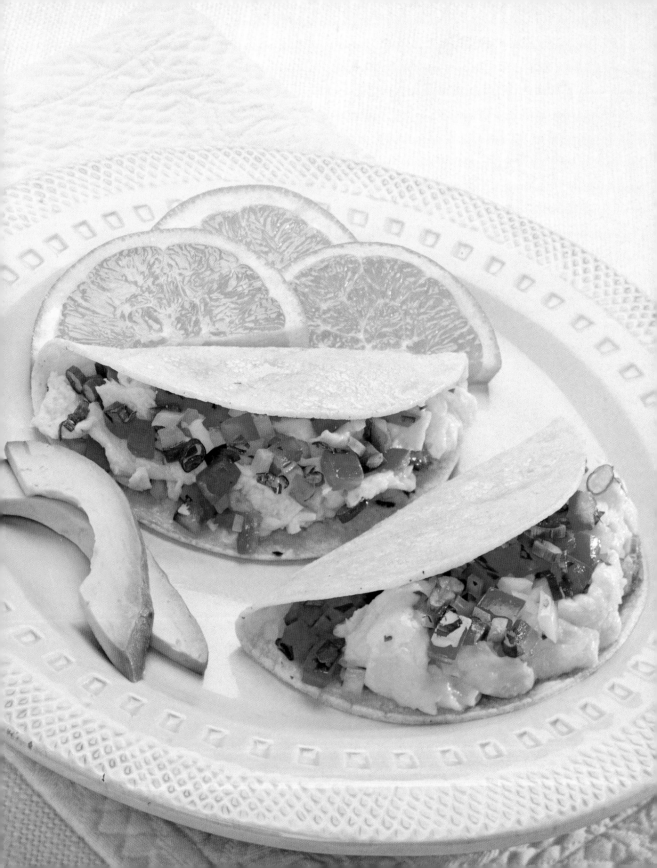

BREAKFAST TACOS

These light, satisfying breakfast tacos bring the flavors of Mexico into your kitchen on even the busiest mornings.

MAKES 4 SERVINGS

Cooking spray
4 large eggs, lightly beaten
4 large egg whites, lightly beaten
2 green onions, sliced (optional)
Eight 6-inch corn tortillas
½ avocado, diced
¾ cup prepared salsa
4 oranges

1. Heat a medium nonstick skillet over medium heat and spray with cooking spray.

2. Add the eggs, egg whites, and green onions, to the skillet and scramble until set, 3 to 4 minutes.

3. Wrap the tortillas in damp paper towels and microwave on high for 1 minute.

4. Divide the eggs evenly among the tortillas and top each with avocado and salsa. Fold into a taco shape.

5. Serve each person two tacos and one orange.

MORE THAN A MELT

What is "more than a melt"? Adding honey ham to this grilled cheese takes it from basic to scrumptious.

MAKES 4 SERVINGS

8 slices whole grain bread
4 teaspoons butter or Better Butter (see page 23)
6 ounces honey ham, thinly sliced
Six 1-ounce slices 2% American cheese
4 slices honeydew melon (⅛ melon each)

1. Preheat broiler.

2. Toast the bread and spread with butter. Place in an oven-safe baking dish large enough to hold all the slices in one layer.

3. Divide the ham evenly on each slice of toast.

4. Top each slice of toast with ¾ slice of American cheese.

5. Place the sandwiches under the broiler to melt the cheese, 1 to 2 minutes.

6. Serve each person two slices of toast with one slice of melon.

BREAKFAST SAUSAGE SANDWICH

Though sausage isn't always thought of as a "lean" meat, turkey sausage is the exception. The average turkey sausage patty has about 15 percent fewer calories and about half the fat of pork sausage. So go ahead and enjoy this guiltless pleasure.

MAKES 4 SERVINGS

8 ounces precooked, frozen turkey sausage patties
2 sourdough English muffins, halved
4 slices tomato
4 ounces shredded part-skim mozzarella, about ½ cup
¼ teaspoon dried basil
¼ teaspoon dried oregano

1. Preheat the broiler.

2. Place the turkey patties on a microwave-safe plate and microwave until defrosted, 1 to 2 minutes.

3. Toast the English muffins and place in an oven-safe baking dish large enough to hold them in one layer.

4. Place one slice of tomato on each muffin half. Divide the sausages evenly among the four muffins and top each with 2 tablespoons shredded cheese. Sprinkle with basil and oregano.

5. Place the English muffins under the broiler and cook until the cheese is melted, 2 to 3 minutes.

6. Serve each person one English muffin half.

SOY BREAKFAST BURRITO

This meatless breakfast burrito will give you a spicy reason to get out of bed in the morning. Soy crumbles, creamy cheese, and hot salsa make a burrito so delicious that you'll never miss the meat.

MAKES 4 SERVINGS

Cooking spray
8 ounces soy crumbles
1 cup prepared salsa
4 ounces shredded Monterey Jack cheese, about ½ cup
Four 10-inch flour tortillas
1 avocado, pitted and sliced
2 tablespoons fat-free sour cream
2 cups cubed mango

1. Spray a nonstick skillet with cooking spray and heat over medium heat.

2. Add the soy crumbles and ½ cup salsa and cook until heated through, 3 to 4 minutes.

3. Wrap the tortillas in damp paper towels and microwave for 1 minute. Remove from the microwave and place one tortilla on each of four plates.

4. Place one-fourth of the soy-salsa mixture on each tortilla. Top with 2 tablespoons cheese. Roll into a burrito shape.

5. Serve each person one burrito topped with the remaining salsa, avocado, and ½ tablespoon sour cream. Serve with ½ cup of cubed mango.

BREAKFAST SAUSAGE BISCUITS

This hearty breakfast of biscuits, sausage, and cheese will rival your favorite restaurant version. Buy precooked biscuits; they're even quicker to prepare than refrigerator biscuits.

MAKES 4 SERVINGS

4 precooked biscuits or 1 small can refrigerator biscuits (4)
½ pound ground chicken
½ teaspoon poultry seasoning
¼ teaspoon salt
1 teaspoon fennel seeds
¼ teaspoon freshly ground black pepper
Four 1-ounce slices low-fat cheddar cheese
2 cups no-sugar-added pineapple juice

1. Preheat the oven to 425°F. Heat a George Foreman–type grill to medium-high.

2. If using precooked biscuits, place in the oven to warm through, 6 to 7 minutes. If using refrigerated biscuits, bake according to package instructions.

3. Combine the chicken, poultry seasoning, salt, fennel, and pepper in a large bowl. Mix until thoroughly combined and form into four patties.

4. Place the patties on the bottom of the grill. Close the top and grill until cooked through and no pink remains, 4 to 5 minutes.

5. Halve the biscuits. Place a chicken patty on each bottom half. Top with one slice of cheese and the other half of the biscuit.

6. Serve each person one biscuit with ½ cup pineapple juice.

HAM AND RICOTTA PITA

Ricotta, an Italian cheese made from the whey that results when making cheeses such as mozzarella and provolone, is similar in texture, though considerably lighter, than cottage cheese. However, if you prefer cottage cheese, feel free to substitute, but make sure you choose a low-fat variety.

MAKES 4 SERVINGS

1 cup part-skim ricotta cheese
4 ounces shredded part-skim mozzarella cheese, about ½ cup
1 teaspoon dried oregano
1 teaspoon dried basil
2 whole pita pocket breads, halved
4 ounces thinly sliced lean ham, cut into strips
Four 8-ounce glasses skim milk

1. Preheat the oven to 425°F.

2. Stir together the ricotta, mozzarella, oregano, and basil in a medium bowl. Place ¼ cup cheese mixture into each pita pocket half and top with ham. Wrap in foil and place in the oven for 5 to 6 minutes or until heated through.

3. Serve each person one pita pocket half with one glass of milk.

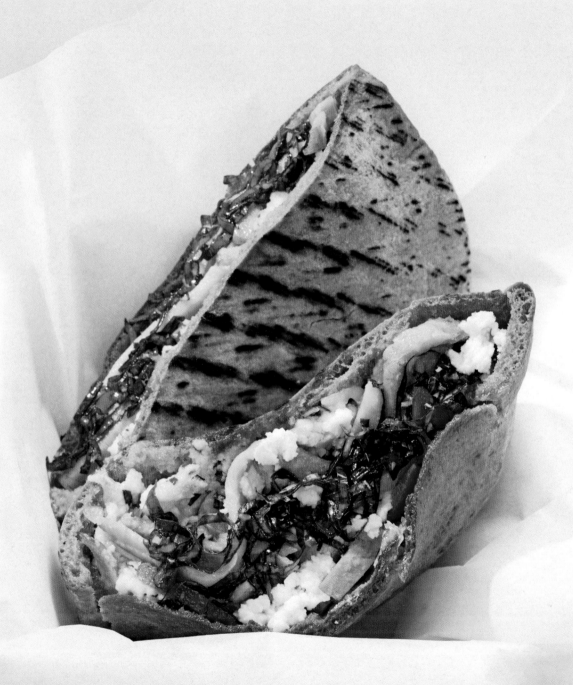

BUBBLING CINNAMON TOAST

Make this sweet, rich-tasting breakfast and your kitchen will be filled with the heady aroma of cinnamon and apples. Wash it down with skim milk.

MAKES 4 SERVINGS

Cooking spray
4 slices cinnamon bread, cubed
2 cups egg substitute, such as Egg Beaters®
2 teaspoons cinnamon
6 tablespoons reduced-fat cream cheese, softened
2 cups unsweetened applesauce
Four 8-ounce glasses skim milk

1. Heat a large nonstick skillet over medium heat and spray with cooking spray.

2. Layer the bread cubes in skillet and pour egg substitute over the bread cubes. Sprinkle with cinnamon, and cook, covered, until set, 5 to 6 minutes.

3. Slice into four portions and top each portion with 1½ tablespoons cream cheese and ½ cup applesauce.

4. Serve each portion with a glass of milk.

CHEDDAR STRATA MELT

Generally considered a brunch entreé, strata is a classic Italian dish made with various ingredients layered over a base of day-old bread and fresh cheeses. This version includes a flavorful array of cheeses, including cheddar, ricotta, and Parmesan.

MAKES 4 SERVINGS

4 slices whole grain bread
8 ounces shredded cheddar cheese, about 1 cup
1 cup nonfat ricotta cheese
4 tablespoons grated Parmesan
4 small peaches

1. Preheat the broiler. Line a baking sheet with aluminum foil.

2. Toast the bread and place in a single layer on the baking sheet.

3. Mix together the cheddar, ricotta, and Parmesan in a small bowl. Divide evenly and spread on each piece of toast.

4. Broil the toast until the cheese bubbles, 2 to 3 minutes.

5. Serve each person one slice of strata with one peach.

RICOTTA CHEESE TOAST

Here's a combination that you will find quickly replaces plain old toast and jam. Broiled ricotta cheese mixed with apricot, cinnamon, and nutmeg and topped with mandarin oranges makes this a delectable morning treat.

MAKES 4 SERVINGS

Eight ½-inch-thick slices French bread
Cooking spray
2 cups part-skim ricotta cheese
2 tablespoons dried apricots, chopped
1 teaspoon cinnamon
¼ teaspoon nutmeg
1 cup mandarin oranges canned in juice, drained, reserving 1 tablespoon juice
Four 8-ounce glasses skim milk

1. Preheat the broiler.

2. Spray the bread with nonstick cooking spray and place on a cookie sheet. Broil until toasted, turning once, 2 to 3 minutes total.

3. Mix the ricotta cheese with apricots, cinnamon, nutmeg, and the reserved juice from oranges. Spread ¼ cup cheese mixture on each piece of toast.

4. Broil toast until cheese mixture turns light brown, 1 minute. Top with mandarin oranges.

5. Serve each person two pieces of toast with one glass of milk.

MOZZARELLA AND TOMATO ON TOASTED ONION ROLL

Did you know that onions can lower your cholesterol and blood pressure? Yep, onions contain sulfur compounds, which account for their pungent smell, as well as chromium and vitamin B_6. These vitamins and minerals lower homocysteine levels in the blood, which decreases your risk of heart attack and stroke.

MAKES 4 SERVINGS

4 onion rolls
8 slices red onion
8 slices tomato
8 ounces shredded nonfat mozzarella, about 1 cup
Four 6-ounce glasses skim milk
4 small plums

1. Preheat the broiler or toaster oven.

2. Slice each onion roll in half and lightly toast under the broiler.

3. Top each onion roll half with one slice of red onion, one slice of tomato, and 1 ounce (2 tablespoons) cheese.

4. Place under the broiler until cheese just melts, 45 seconds to 1 minute.

5. Serve each person two halves of an onion roll with a glass of milk and a plum.

FRUITY PIZZA

Pizza doesn't have to be laden with fattening meat and cheese to be delicious. Our breakfast pizza, made with low-fat cream cheese and fresh fruit, is sweet and tasty. Garnish these pizzas with fresh mint for an attractive presentation.

MAKES 4 SERVINGS

Four 6-inch pocketless pita breads
4 tablespoons low-fat cream cheese
2 cups low-fat cottage cheese
½ cup mixed berries
4 peaches, sliced (about 1 pound)
½ teaspoon cinnamon
2 tablespoons sliced almonds
Four 6-ounce glasses skim milk

1. Spread each pita with 1 tablespoon cream cheese, and then with ½ cup cottage cheese.

2. Top each pita with berries and peaches, dividing the fruit equally. Sprinkle with cinnamon and sliced almonds.

3. Serve each person one pita with a glass of milk.

STUFFED PANCAKES

Top these protein-rich pancakes with cherries, which have several health benefits. For example, the cherries' red pigment, called anthocyanin, has been shown to reduce pain and inflammation.

MAKES 4 SERVINGS

8 frozen pancakes
1 cup part-skim ricotta cheese
3 cups 1% cottage cheese
2 cups pitted cherries (thawed if frozen, drained if canned)
Four 6-ounce glasses skim milk

1. Heat the pancakes in a toaster according to the package instructions.

2. Mix together the ricotta and cottage cheese in a bowl.

3. Top each pancake with ¼ cup cheese mixture and ¼ cup cherries.

4. Serve each person two pancakes and one glass of milk.

WAFFLE WITH COTTAGE CHEESE AND FRUIT

Cottage cheese is an excellent source of protein and calcium. A half cup, for example, supplies as much protein as 2 ounces of cooked lean beef, fish, or chicken as well as 100 mg of calcium.

MAKES 4 SERVINGS

4 whole grain frozen waffles
3 cups nonfat cottage cheese
1½ teaspoons Barlean's® organic flaxseed oil
2 bananas, sliced
1 cup mixed berries (thawed if frozen)
4 tablespoons chopped peanuts
Four 6-ounce glasses skim milk

1. Toast the waffles according to the package instructions. Place one waffle on each of four plates.

2. Mix the cottage cheese with flaxseed oil in a small bowl.

3. Spread one-fourth of the cottage cheese mixture on each waffle and top with bananas, berries, and chopped peanuts.

4. Serve each person one waffle with one glass of milk.

OATS WITH TURKEY BACON

A substantial and comforting food choice, oatmeal can help reduce the risk of heart disease when combined with a low-fat diet.

MAKES 4 SERVINGS

8 slices turkey bacon
4 cups low-fat milk or low-fat soy milk
1½ cups rolled oats
2 cups blueberries (thawed if frozen)
½ cup slivered almonds
3 tablespoons maple syrup

1. Heat a nonstick skillet over medium heat.

2. Add the turkey bacon and sauté until crisp, 3 minutes, turning frequently.

3. Bring the milk to a boil in a medium saucepan over medium heat. Stir in the oats. Bring the mixture back to a boil and reduce heat. Simmer until the oatmeal is tender and has absorbed most of the milk, 8 minutes.

4. Portion into four bowls and add equal amounts of blueberries, almonds, and maple syrup to each bowl. Serve with two slices of turkey bacon on the side.

BREAKFAST BANANA SPLIT

Wheat germ is the embryo of a wheat kernel that's usually removed before milling into cereal, which is a shame. Wheat germ contains more nutrients per ounce than any other grain or vegetable. It contains large amounts of protein, iron, potassium, B vitamins, and vitamin E, among many others. In addition to these health benefits, wheat germ has a wonderful nutty flavor.

MAKES 4 SERVINGS

4 cups nonfat vanilla yogurt
2 teaspoons Barlean's® organic flaxseed oil
4 small, ripe bananas
4 tablespoons peanut butter
6 tablespoons wheat germ
Four 6-ounce glasses skim milk

1. Mix together the yogurt and flaxseed oil in a medium bowl.

2. Split each banana in half lengthwise and place two halves on each of four plates.

3. Spread each banana half with ½ tablespoon peanut butter.

4. Top with the yogurt mixture and sprinkle with wheat germ.

5. Serve each person one banana split with a glass milk.

BAKED CINNAMON APPLE WITH COTTAGE CHEESE AND WALNUTS

Fill your kitchen with the warm, comforting aroma of baked apples with this mouthwatering breakfast entrée.

MAKES 4 SERVINGS

2 large apples, sliced
4 teaspoons cinnamon
2 teaspoons Barlean's® organic flaxseed oil
4 cups nonfat cottage cheese
2 tablespoons honey
4 tablespoons chopped walnuts
Four 6-ounce glasses skim milk

1. Place the apples in a microwave-safe container and sprinkle with 2 teaspoons cinnamon. Microwave until soft, turning occasionally, 3 minutes.

2. Stir the flaxseed oil into cottage cheese.

3. Divide the cottage cheese mixture among four plates and top with the apples.

4. Drizzle with the honey and sprinkle with walnuts and the remaining cinnamon.

5. Serve each person one plate with a glass of milk.

Instant Meals

The most important meal of the day, breakfast, is often the hardest to get people to eat. They just don't have time to prepare a meal in the morning, even if it only takes 10 minutes! That's why I created the following "Instant Meals." These recipes are for those mornings when you hardly have time to brush your teeth, let alone eat breakfast. They require no cooking and are ready in no time. Now, you have no reason not to start your day feeling fed, satisfied, and ready to take on the world!

BREAKFAST HAM AND CHEESE

A simple classic, such as a ham and cheese sandwich, makes a quick and easy breakfast. Served with fresh fruit, it's a delicious and satisfying way to start your day.

MAKES 4 SERVINGS

8 slices whole grain bread
4 tablespoons Dijon mustard
8 thin slices lean deli ham
Four 1-ounce slices Swiss cheese
4 apples

1. Toast bread. Spread each slice of bread with ½ tablespoon mustard.

2. Layer two slices of ham and one slice of cheese on each of four slices of bread. Top with the remaining slices of bread.

3. Serve each person one sandwich with one apple.

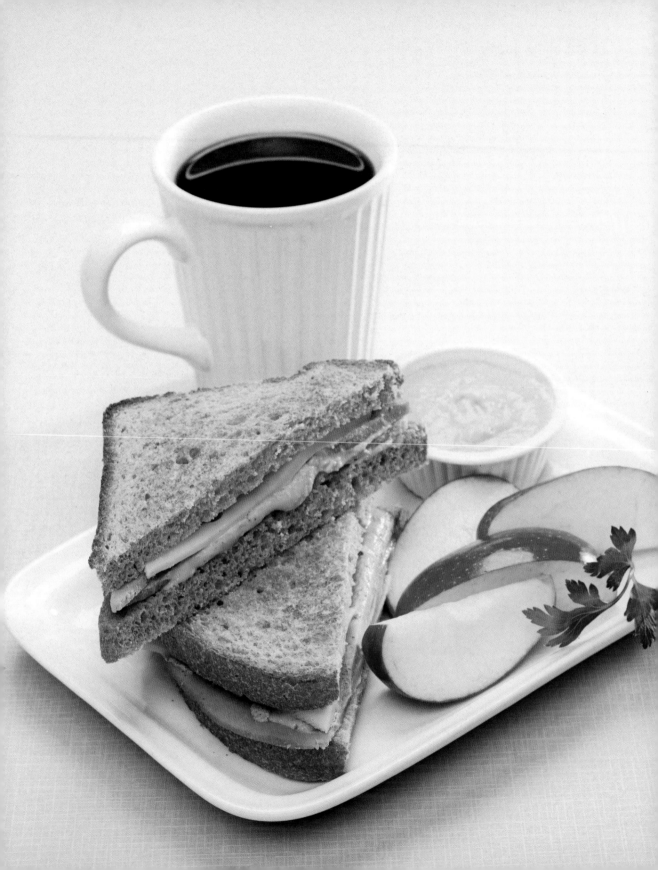

BREAKFAST BURRITO

It won't get much quicker than this meal. Enjoy a simple and easy breakfast burrito when you just don't have any time to spend making breakfast.

MAKES 4 SERVINGS

4 Amy's® frozen Breakfast Burritos
½ avocado, sliced into 8 pieces
4 cups sliced strawberries

1. Heat the burritos in a microwave oven according to the package instructions.

2. Top each burrito with two slices of avocado.

3. Serve each person one burrito with 1 cup strawberries.

ALMOND BUTTER AND BANANA TOAST

Bananas are not only packed with potassium, but they're also a tasty way to start your day. Pair them with almonds and flaxseed oil, both of which contain heart-healthy fats, and you have a delicious and nourishing breakfast.

MAKES 4 SERVINGS

1 tablespoon Barlean's® organic flaxseed oil
7 tablespoons almond butter
8 slices whole grain bread
2 medium bananas, sliced

1. Toast the bread.

2. In a small bowl, stir the flaxseed oil into the almond butter.

3. Spread 1 tablespoon almond butter mixture on each slice of toast.

4. Top with the sliced banana.

5. Serve each person two slices of toast.

PEANUT BUTTER AND BANANA

Adding wheat germ to this fabulously simple toast, peanut butter, and banana concoction gives it a concentrated source of essential nutrients, including folic acid, phosphorous, thiamine, zinc, and magnesium.

MAKES 4 SERVINGS

4 slices whole grain bread
8 tablespoons peanut butter
2 bananas, sliced
4 tablespoons wheat germ
Four 6-ounce glasses skim milk

1. Toast the bread.

2. Spread each slice of toast with 2 tablespoons peanut butter.

3. Top each slice of toast with half of a sliced banana and 1 tablespoon wheat germ.

4. Serve each person one slice of peanut butter toast and a glass of milk.

TOAST WITH ALMOND BUTTER AND COTTAGE CHEESE

Almond butter is a delicious alternative to peanut butter for those with peanut allergies or who just want a change of pace. Serve with cups of steaming herbal tea for a satisfying, invigorating breakfast.

MAKES 4 SERVINGS

1½ teaspoons Barlean's® organic flaxseed oil
4 tablespoons almond butter
4 slices whole grain bread
3 cups nonfat cottage cheese
2 cups diced pineapple (thawed if frozen, drained if canned)

1. In a small bowl, stir together the flaxseed oil and almond butter.

2. Toast the bread and spread with 1 tablespoon almond butter mixture.

3. In a separate bowl, combine the cottage cheese and pineapple.

4. Serve each person one slice of almond toast and one-fourth of the cottage cheese-pineapple mixture.

WAFFLES WITH ALMOND BUTTER

You'll find everyone satisfied with this meal of waffles and almond butter. Shop for whole grain waffles, which are nutritionally superior to refined-grain waffles.

MAKES 4 SERVINGS

4 whole grain frozen waffles
4 tablespoons almond butter
2 bananas, sliced
Four 8-ounce glasses 1% milk

1. Toast the waffles according to the package instructions.

2. Top each toasted waffle with 1 tablespoon almond butter and half of a sliced banana.

2. Serve each person one waffle with one glass of milk.

COTTAGE CHEESE WITH GRANOLA AND FRESH FRUIT

Colorful and savory, this crunchy breakfast looks beautiful in a clear parfait glass.

MAKES 4 SERVINGS

2 teaspoons Barlean's® organic flaxseed oil
3 cups nonfat cottage cheese
3 cups mixed berries (thawed if frozen)
2 cups low-fat granola

1. In a small bowl, stir the flaxseed oil into cottage cheese.

2. Using equal amounts, layer the cottage cheese mixture, berries, and granola in four parfait glasses and serve.

CEREAL WITH MILK AND COTTAGE CHEESE

You've heard of cereal, cottage cheese, and milk, but have you ever tried quark? Quark is a relatively modern, soft, spreadable cheese with a very low fat content. It has a slightly tangy flavor that's similar to low-fat ricotta. Try it in place of cottage cheese in this recipe for a change of pace.

MAKES 4 SERVINGS

4 cups Kashi GOLEAN® Crunch! Cereal
4 cups skim milk or fat-free soy milk
2 cups blueberries (thawed if frozen)
2 cups nonfat cottage cheese or quark
1 teaspoon Barlean's® organic flaxseed oil

1. Divide the cereal among four bowls and add 1 cup of milk per bowl.

2. Mix the blueberries and flaxseed oil into the cottage cheese or quark. Divide equally among four smaller bowls.

3. Serve each person one bowl of cereal and one bowl of the cottage cheese mixture.

MUESLI AND FRUIT

Muesli is a Swiss cereal that typically includes rolled oats, nuts, seeds, and a variety of dried fruits. There are several varieties on the market, but you can easily make your own. Experiment with different grains, nuts, and fruits to create your own unique concoction.

MAKES 4 SERVINGS

2 cups muesli
2 cups nonfat vanilla yogurt
1 teaspoon Barlean's® organic flaxseed oil
8 tablespoons raw almonds, chopped
2 cups raspberries (thawed if frozen)

1. Mix all the ingredients together in a bowl.

2. Divide equally into four bowls and serve.

Chapter 5

YOGURT, SHAKES & SMOOTHIES

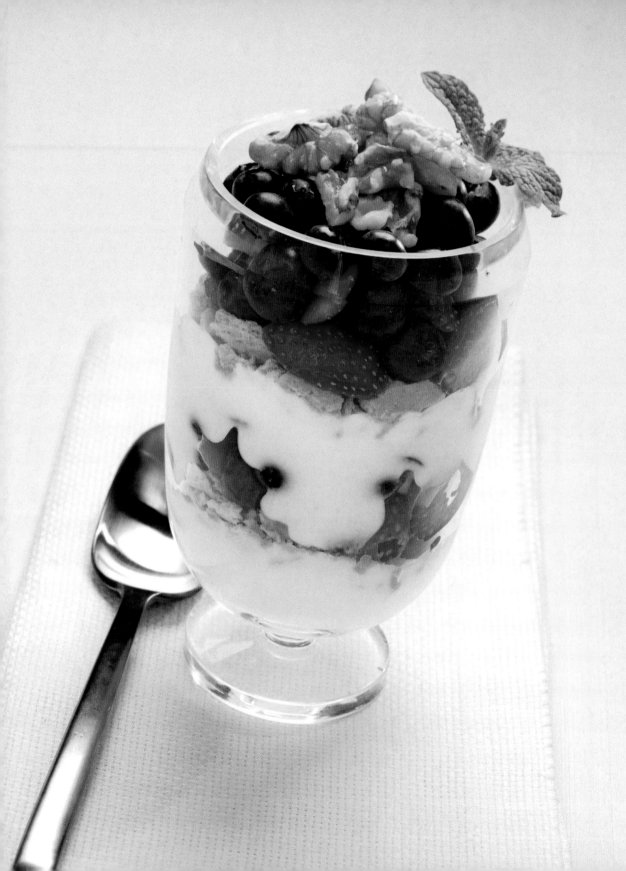

VANILLA YOGURT AND BERRY PARFAIT

This tasty yogurt-berry delight will give you energy to get through a challenging morning. You can also serve it as a fancy, colorful brunch on a special weekend morning.

MAKES 4 SERVINGS

3 cups low-fat vanilla yogurt
1 tablespoon lemon juice (optional)
1½ cups raspberries (thawed if frozen)
1½ cups blackberries (thawed if frozen)
1 cup Grape-Nuts cereal

1. In a small bowl, stir together the yogurt and lemon juice, if using.

2. In another small bowl, gently mix together the raspberries and blackberries, reserving four raspberries and four blackberries for garnish.

3. Layer ½ cup berries into each of four parfait glasses. Top with ½ cup yogurt mixture. Top each with ¼ cup berries and the remaining yogurt.

4. Top each parfait with ¼ cup cereal and the reserved berries.

5. Serve each person one parfait.

SOY CRANBERRY SHAKE WITH PEANUT BUTTER TOAST

Getting to know soy is not as challenging as it may seem. Soy milk comes in nonfat, low-fat, and flavored varieties. Try substituting vanilla-flavored soy milk for the plain variety in this shake.

MAKES 4 SERVINGS

2 cups low-fat soy milk
1 cup low-fat vanilla yogurt
1⅓ cups cranberry juice
½ teaspoon vanilla extract
1 teaspoon cinnamon
4 slices whole grain bread
2 tablespoons peanut butter

1. Combine the soy milk, yogurt, juice, vanilla, and cinnamon in a blender and mix on high speed until well blended. Divide equally among four glasses.

2. Toast the bread.

3. Spread ½ tablespoon peanut butter on each piece of toast.

4. Serve each person one shake and one slice of toast.

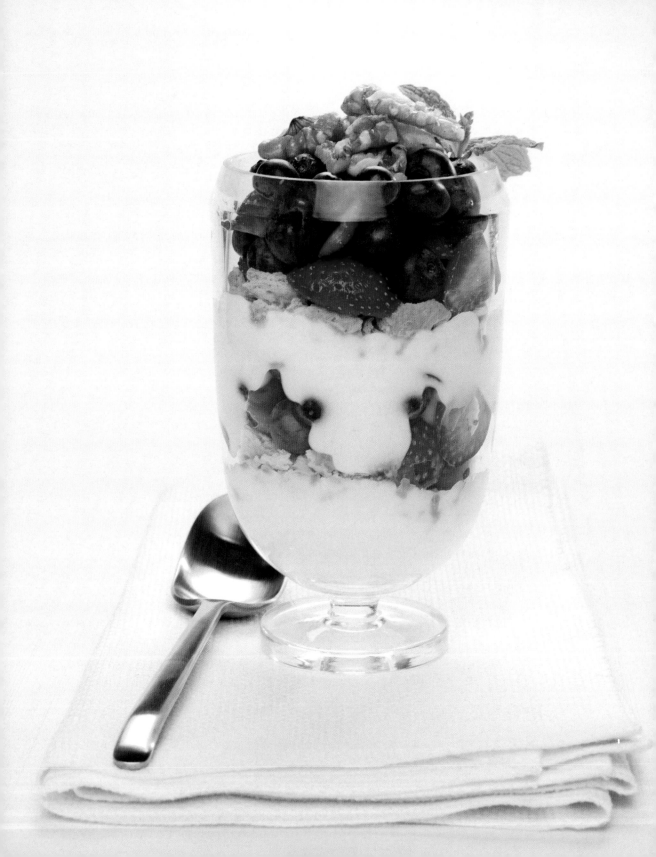

LAYERED YOGURT PARFAIT

Parfait means "perfect" in French, and that's what this meal is. Serve this sweet and crunchy layered treat in a tall, clear glass so that all the food is visible.

MAKES 4 SERVINGS

1 quart low-fat vanilla yogurt
12 squares graham crackers, crushed
1 cup sliced strawberries (thawed if frozen)
1 cup blueberries (thawed if frozen)
¼ cup chopped nuts
Four 6-ounce glasses skim milk

1. Spoon 4 ounces of yogurt into each of four large parfait glasses.

2. Top with half of the graham crackers and berries.

3. Repeat with a second layer of yogurt, graham crackers, and berries.

4. Sprinkle with nuts.

5. Serve each person one parfait with one glass of milk.

APPLES, WALNUTS, AND YOGURT

This appetizing meal is packed with nutritional value. Apples provide fiber and antioxidants, and yogurt provides calcium and nonfat protein. In addition, flaxseed oil and walnuts are excellent sources of omega-3 fatty acids, which are helpful in lowering cholesterol.

MAKES 4 SERVINGS

4 medium apples, sliced
2 cups nonfat vanilla yogurt
1½ teaspoons Barlean's organic flaxseed oil
2 teaspoons cinnamon
4 ounces walnuts, chopped, about 1 cup

1.   Divide the sliced apples among four bowls.

2.   Stir together the yogurt, flaxseed oil, cinnamon, and walnuts in a small bowl.

3.   Top each of the four bowls of apples with the yogurt mixture.

4.   Serve each person one bowl.

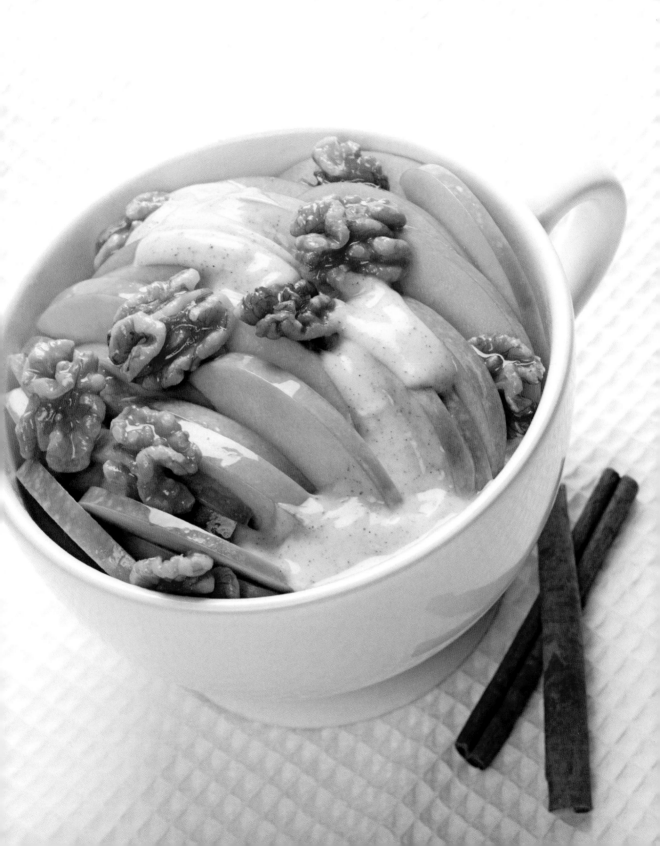

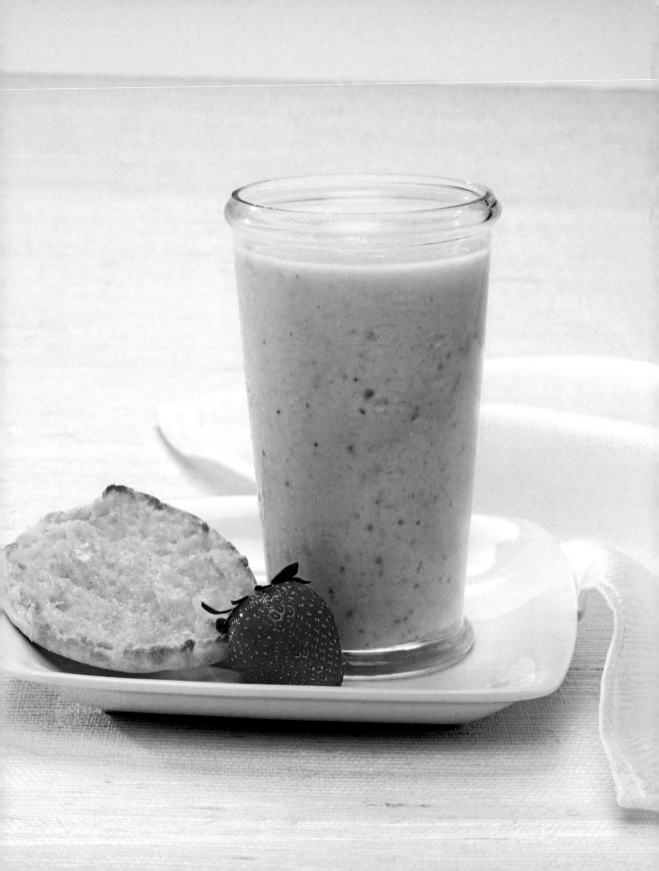

STRAWBERRY-BANANA YOGURT SHAKE

Frozen strawberries in this banana yogurt shake are like sweet, fruity ice cubes, thickening your shake and giving it an extra boost of vitamin C.

MAKES 4 SERVINGS

2 small bananas
1 cup frozen strawberries
2⅔ cups nonfat plain yogurt
1 cup orange juice
2 teaspoons cinnamon
2 whole grain English muffins, halved
4 teaspoons butter or Better Butter (see page 23)

1. Blend the bananas, strawberries, yogurt, and orange juice in a blender until smooth. Pour into four glasses. Sprinkle each with ½ teaspoon of the cinnamon.

2. Toast the English muffins, spread with butter, and sprinkle with the remaining cinnamon.

3. Serve each person one shake and one English muffin half.

ORANGE AND BANANA SMOOTHIE

A special blend of fruit and yogurt, this smoothie is a perfect way to start or end a summer day. Don't forget the sweet almonds, which add healthy fat and contain practically no carbohydrates. Depending on the size of your blender, you may need to make this smoothie in two batches.

MAKES 4 SERVINGS

4 cups vanilla nonfat yogurt
2 teaspoons Barlean's® organic flaxseed oil
4 tablespoons protein powder or skim milk powder (optional)
2 bananas
2 cups orange juice
6 ice cubes
½ cup almonds

1. In a blender, combine the yogurt, flaxseed oil, protein powder (if using), bananas, orange juice, and ice cubes and blend until smooth.

2. Divide the smoothie equally among four glasses and serve with almonds (10 per person).

BREAKFAST SMOOTHIE

Very ripe bananas are the key to sweetening this breakfast smoothie. Experiment with different fruits to find your favorite mixture. Blend this smoothie in two batches if all the ingredients don't fit in your blender carafe.

MAKES 4 SERVINGS

2 cups low-fat milk
2 cups nonfat vanilla yogurt
1 teaspoon Barlean's® organic flaxseed oil
2 cups ice cubes
2 ripe bananas
2 cups frozen fruit of your choice
1 teaspoon vanilla
½ teaspoon cinnamon

1. Combine all the ingredients in a blender and blend until smooth.

2. Divide the smoothie evenly among four glasses and serve.

FLAT BELLY SHAKE

My Flat Belly Shake helps reduce what I call "false fat"—the air, fluid, and waste that can get trapped in your belly when you don't eat enough fiber. Enjoy this shake three times a week as a meal (breakfast, lunch, or dinner), and it will help you shed up to three inches off your belly in one month. Be aware that even though the ingredients take up so much space in the blender, this recipe only serves one.

MAKES 1 SERVING

½ cup ice
½ cup Kashi GOLEAN® Crunch! cereal
1 cup skim milk
1 cup frozen blueberries or another berry of your choice
1 tablespoon psyllium husk powder (available at any health food store)
1 tablespoon Barlean's® organic flaxseed oil

1. Combine all the ingredients in a blender and blend until smooth.

2. Pour into a tall glass and serve.

Chapter 6
PASTA & PIZZA

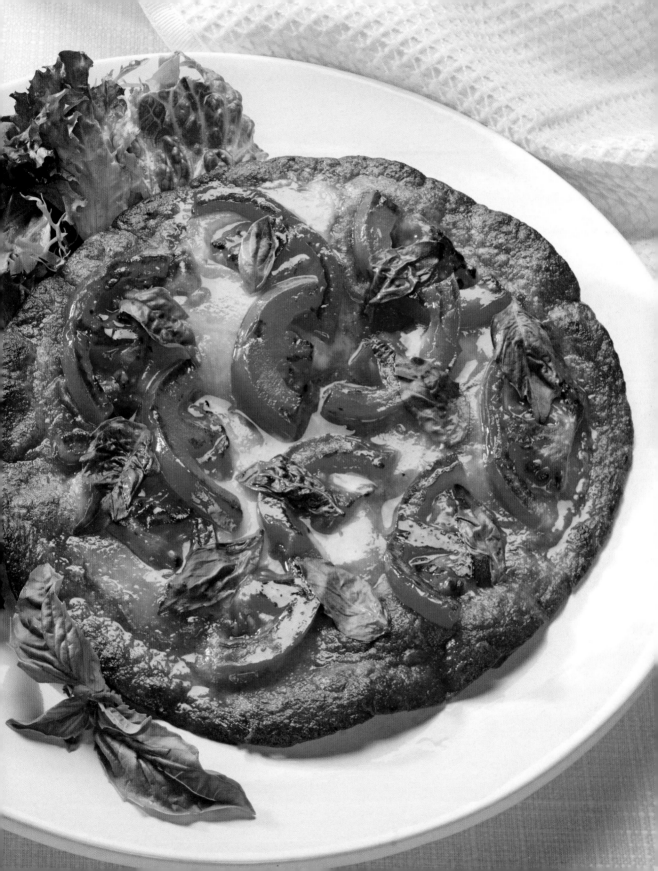

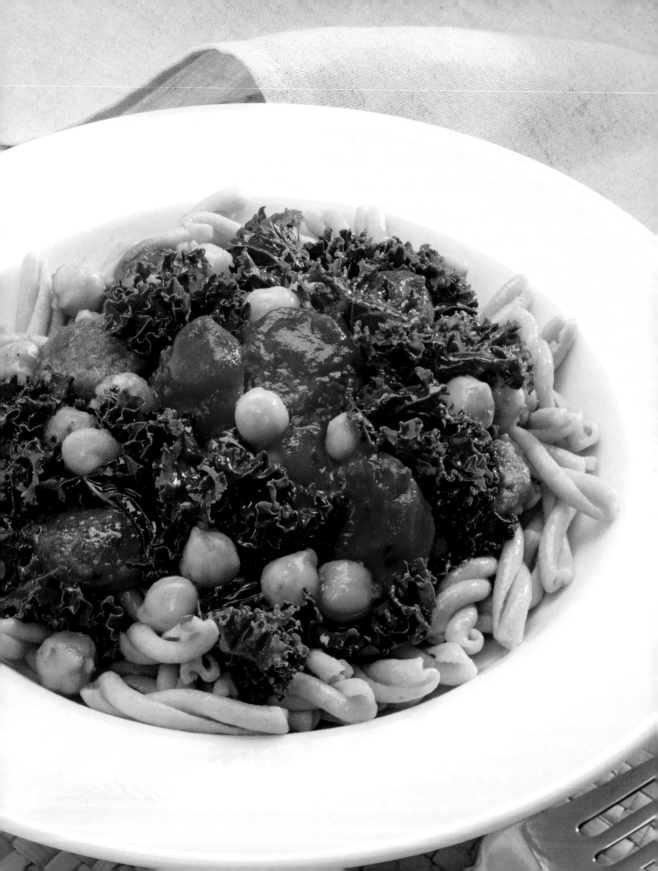

TURKEY SAUSAGE PASTA WITH KALE

Kale belongs to the same family of vegetables as cabbage, collard greens, and Brussels sprouts. Kale is a nutritional powerhouse, high in fiber, and vitamins A, B, and C, and low in calories. Kale also has many cancer-fighting agents called organosulfur compounds. Kale is delicious mixed into pasta and other foods or boiled and eaten as a side dish. It can taste slightly bitter, however, so try pairing it with something sweet, like caramelized onions, for a more balanced flavor experience.

MAKES 4 SERVINGS

12 ounces whole grain gemelli pasta, about 4 cups
Cooking spray
2 links precooked turkey sausage, sliced
3 cups prepared marinara sauce
1 cup chickpeas, rinsed and drained
3 cups fresh kale, stemmed, rinsed, and roughly chopped

1. Cook the pasta according to the package instructions.

2. Heat a large saucepan over medium heat and spray with cooking spray while the pasta cooks.

3. Add the turkey sausage and cook until lightly browned, 5 to 6 minutes.

4. Add the marinara sauce and chickpeas to the sausage and bring to a low boil. Reduce heat to low.

5. Add the kale and simmer until the kale is soft, 5 minutes.

6. Drain the pasta and add to the sauce. Toss to coat the pasta with the sauce.

7. Divide pasta evenly among four bowls and serve.

FUSILLI PASTA WITH SHRIMP AND ARTICHOKES

Fusilli is corkscrew-shaped pasta; if you can't find it, you can substitute with any short pasta, like penne.

MAKES 4 SERVINGS

6 ounces whole grain fusilli pasta, about 2 cups
1½ tablespoons olive oil
½ cup chopped onion
2 tablespoons minced garlic
¾ teaspoon red pepper flakes
1 cup low-sodium chicken broth
2 cups frozen chopped broccoli, thawed
¾ pound cooked shrimp (thawed if frozen)
One 15-ounce can artichoke hearts in water, drained and quartered
¼ cup sliced black olives
½ teaspoon salt
¼ teaspoon pepper

1. Cook the pasta according to the package instructions.

2. Meanwhile, heat a large nonstick skillet over medium-high heat and add the oil, onion, garlic and red pepper flakes. Sauté for 2 to 3 minutes.

3. Add the chicken broth and broccoli. Cover and simmer until the broccoli is tender, 3 to 4 minutes.

4. Stir in the shrimp, artichokes, and olives and cook until heated through, 2 minutes. Season with salt and pepper.

5. Drain the pasta and add to the sauce, tossing to coat.

6. Divide into four equal portions and serve.

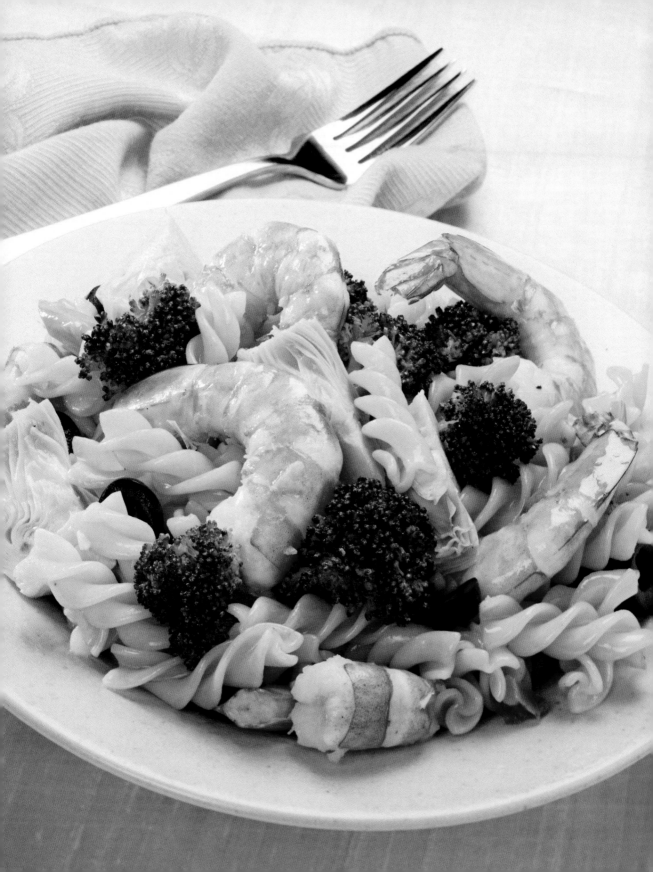

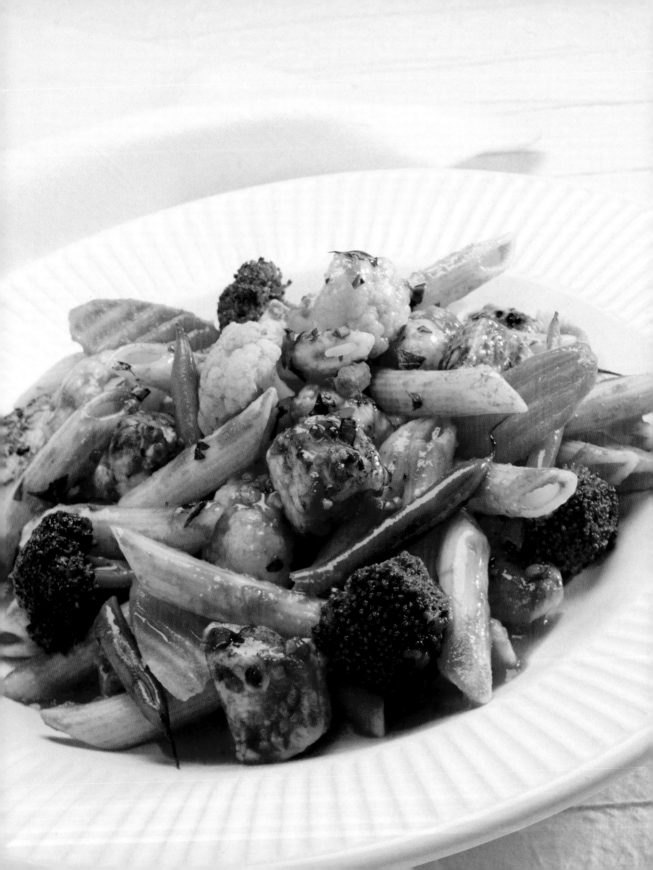

PENNE PASTA WITH CHICKEN AND MIXED VEGGIES

Using frozen vegetables instead of fresh in this dish will save you a lot of time, because they're already cooked. If you want to use fresh veggies, briefly steam or blanch them before adding them to the sauce.

MAKES 4 SERVINGS

9 ounces penne pasta, about 3 cups
1 tablespoon olive oil
1 tablespoon minced garlic
1 pound boneless, skinless chicken breast, cut into 1-inch cubes.
12 ounces frozen vegetable blend, thawed
1 cup prepared marinara sauce

1. Cook the pasta according to the package instructions.

2. Heat a large nonstick skillet over medium-high heat and add the oil.

3. Add the garlic to the skillet and sauté until fragrant, 30 seconds. Add the chicken; cook and stir until no pink remains, 5 minutes.

4. Add the vegetables and marinara sauce and cook until heated through, 6 to 7 minutes.

5. Add the penne to the sauce and toss to coat.

6. Divide the pasta evenly among four bowls and serve.

TOMATO SAUCE OVER LINGUINI WITH TUNA AND CAPERS

Tuna is packed with omega-3 fatty acids, which improve cardiovascular health and reduce the risk for heart disease. Canned in water, it's an excellent source of low-fat protein.

MAKES 4 SERVINGS

6 ounces linguine
1 tablespoon olive oil
1 medium red onion, chopped
2 cups prepared marinara sauce
1 tablespoon capers, drained
Two 6-ounce pouches or cans water-packed tuna
¼ cup sliced black olives
1 tablespoon grated lemon peel
½ teaspoon salt
¼ teaspoon black pepper
4 cups mixed salad greens
⅓ cup thinly sliced red onion
½ cup fat-free vinaigrette

1. Cook the linguine according to the package instructions.

2. While the pasta cooks, heat a large nonstick skillet over medium heat and add the oil.

3. Add the onion to the skillet and sauté for 3 to 4 minutes.

4. Add the sauce, capers, tuna, olives, and lemon peel. Bring to a boil and reduce heat to low. Stir in the salt and black pepper.

5. Drain the pasta and add to the sauce. Toss to coat.

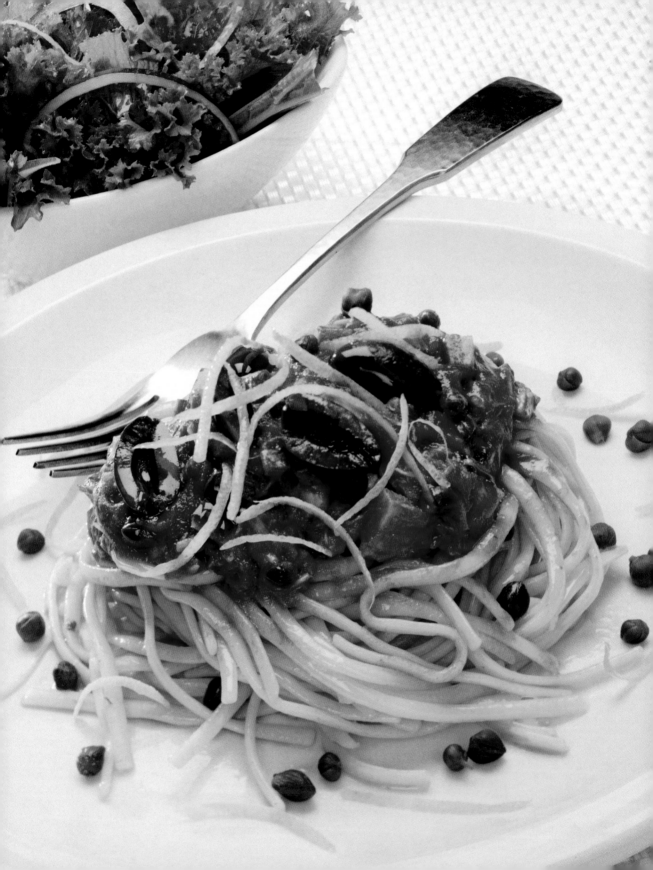

6.   Combine the salad greens and onion in a large bowl. Add the vinaigrette and toss to coat. Divide among four salad plates.

7.   Divide the pasta into four equal portions and serve with the salad.

TURKEY AND SPINACH LASAGNA

I made this lasagna with my good friend Emeril Lagasse on his cooking show, Emeril LIVE!. It's a delicious example of how you can get your protein, carbs, and veggies in one dish. This lasagna makes 12 servings, unlike the other recipes in this book, so make sure to save your leftovers for lunch the next day. Also, this recipe takes a bit longer to make than some of the others, but it's well worth the effort!

MAKES 12 SERVINGS

8 whole wheat lasagna noodles
1 tablespoon olive oil
½ cup chopped onion
1 chopped bell pepper, any color
1½ pounds ground hot Italian turkey sausage
6 garlic cloves, chopped
3½ cups prepared marinara sauce
3 cups shredded part-skim mozzarella cheese, divided
1½ cups part-skim ricotta
½ cup crumbled goat cheese
2 cups chopped frozen spinach, thawed and drained
¼ cup grated Parmesan cheese
1 egg, lightly beaten
¼ cup chopped fresh basil
¼ cup chopped fresh parsley

¼ cup chopped fresh oregano
¼ teaspoon black pepper
¼ teaspoon salt

1. Preheat oven to 350°F.

2. Bring several quarts of salted water to a boil in a large pot. Add noodles and cook until tender, 7 minutes. Remove from water and place on a towel-lined baking sheet.

3. Place the olive oil, onion, and bell pepper in a large sauté pan over medium high heat. Sauté until the vegetables begin to sweat, 5 minutes.

4. Add sausage and garlic and and stir to combine. Sauté until sausage cooks through, 10 minutes.

5. Add pasta sauce to sausage mixture and bring to a boil. Reduce heat to low and simmer 10 minutes. Remove from heat.

6. In a large bowl, combine 1½ cups mozzarella and remaining ingredients; set aside.

7. To assemble: Spray a 13 x 9–inch baking dish with cooking spray. Spread 1 cup sausage mixture in the bottom of the dish and arrange 4 noodles over the turkey mixture; top with 1½ cups sausage mixture. Spread half of the cheese mixture over sausage mixture. Repeat layers, ending with the remaining sausage mixture. Sprinkle with remaining 1½ cups mozzarella cheese.

8. Bake at 350° for 45 minutes or until the cheese is melted and browned and the lasagna is hot and bubbly.

9. Remove from the oven and let cool for at least 20 minutes. Cut the lasagna into 12 equal pieces. Serve each person one piece of lasagna and reserve the remainder for another meal.

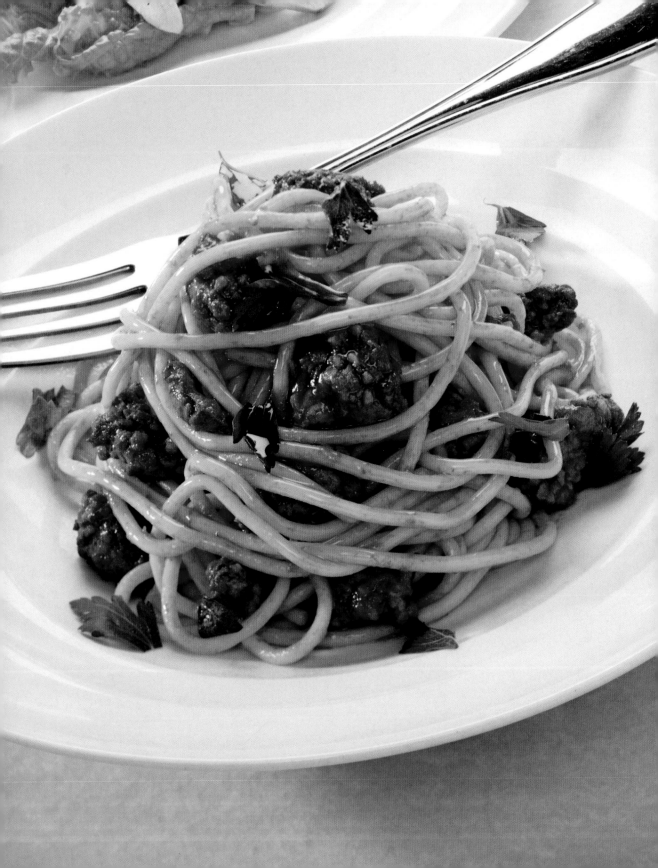

SPAGHETTI WITH MEAT SAUCE AND CAESAR SALAD

This recipe marries the convenience of jarred pasta sauce with freshly cooked beef and chopped herbs. As the sauce cooks, your kitchen will fill with the intoxicating aroma of an Italian restaurant.

MAKES 4 SERVINGS

12 ounces spaghetti
½ pound extra-lean ground beef
1 tablespoon minced garlic
1 cup prepared marinara sauce
¼ cup chopped fresh herbs such as basil, oregano, and/or parsley
4 cups chopped romaine lettuce
¼ cup low-fat Caesar salad dressing

1. Cook the spaghetti according to the package instructions.

2. Heat a large nonstick skillet over medium heat.

3. Add the beef and garlic to the skillet and cook until beef browns and no pink remains, 6 minutes. Drain off the fat.

4. Add the marinara sauce to the meat and bring to a simmer.

5. Drain the spaghetti and add to the meat sauce. Stir in the herbs and toss to combine.

6. Toss the romaine with the Caesar dressing in a large bowl. Divide equally among four plates.

7. Divide the pasta evenly among four bowls and serve with the salad.

GNOCCHI WITH TURKEY SAUSAGE AND SPINACH

Gnocchi is an Italian dumpling that's made by mixing mashed potatoes with flour to create a dough. These little potato pillows are so tender that they melt in your mouth.

MAKES 4 SERVINGS

2 links turkey Italian sausage
1 pound potato gnocchi
3 cups prepared marinara sauce
2 cups baby spinach
¼ cup chopped fresh herbs, such as thyme, oregano, or parsley
4 apricots

1. Preheat oven to 375°F.

2. Slice the turkey sausage lengthwise without cutting all the way through. Open the sliced sausage like a book and place cut side down on a baking sheet.

3. Roast the sausage in the oven until cooked through, 8 to 10 minutes. Remove from heat and let cool. Slice into 1-inch pieces.

4. Cook the gnocchi according to package instructions. Drain.

5. Heat a large saucepan over medium heat and add the marinara. Bring to a simmer.

6. Add the gnocchi, spinach, herbs, and sliced sausage to the marinara sauce. Bring the sauce back to a simmer.

7. Divide the gnocchi equally among four bowls. Serve each person one bowl of pasta and one apricot.

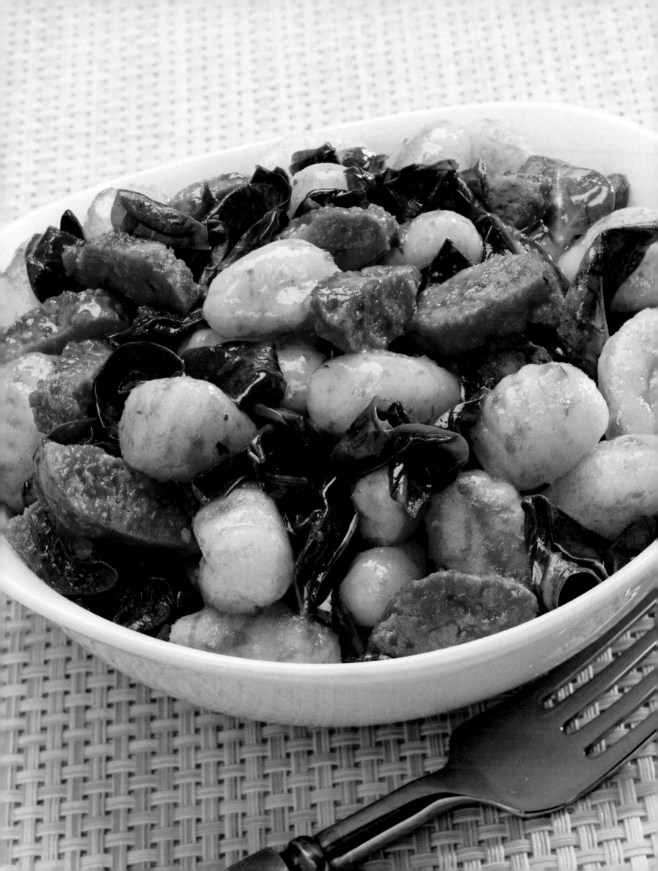

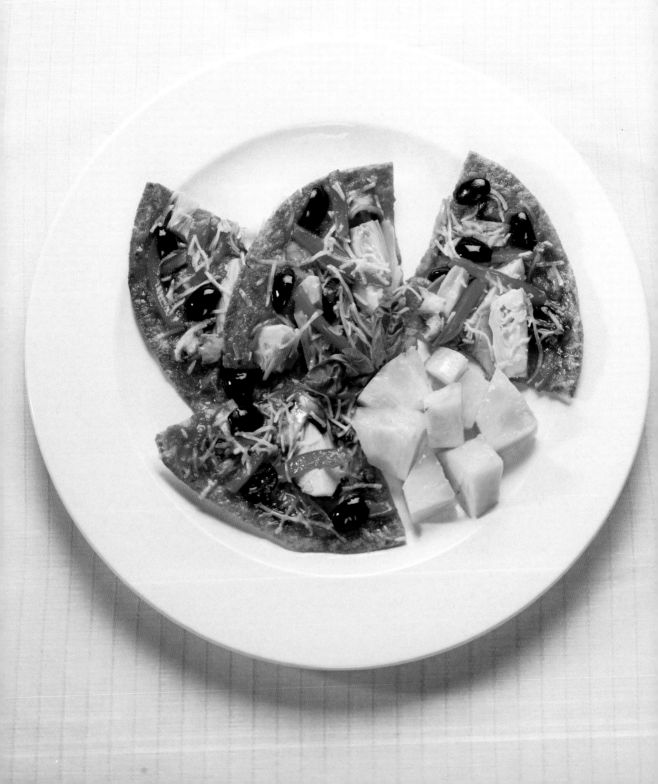

TORTILLA PIZZA

Tomatoes are packed with lycopene, a powerful antioxidant that may reduce the risk of various types of cancer. Research demonstrates that your body absorbs lycopene better when it is in the form of cooked tomato products, such as pizza sauce, rather than raw. Slather this tortilla pizza with plenty of tomato sauce and a enjoy a delicious way to protect your body.

MAKES 4 SERVINGS

Four 10-inch whole wheat tortillas
2 cups prepared pizza sauce
3¼ cup olives, water-packed artichoke hearts, bell peppers, mushrooms, or
     vegetables of your choice, thinly sliced
1 ounce grated Parmesan, about 1 tablespoon
4 cups pineapple cubes (thawed if frozen, drained if canned)

1. Preheat the oven to 400°F. Line a baking sheet with aluminum foil.

2. Place the tortillas on an oven rack and bake until slightly crisp, 5 minutes.

3. Remove the tortillas from the oven and place on the baking sheet.

4. Spread the pizza sauce evenly among the tortillas and top with the vegetables and Parmesan.

5. Bake until vegetables are softened and cheese is melted, 5 to 8 minutes.

6. Serve each person one tortilla pizza with 1 cup of pineapple cubes.

GRILLED CHICKEN, ARTICHOKE, AND GOAT CHEESE PIZZA

Here's a way to use leftover chicken or vegetables that have been taking up space in your refrigerator. You can even add leftover herbs, such as oregano or basil, to make your pizza taste extra fresh.

MAKES 4 SERVINGS

Two 6-inch whole grain pita breads
½ cup prepared marinara sauce
8 ounces cooked chicken breast meat, diced
One 15-ounce can artichokes hearts in water, drained and quartered
4 ounces goat cheese crumbles, about ½ cup

1. Preheat the oven to 375°F. Line a baking sheet with aluminum foil.

2. Place the pitas on the baking sheet and spread each pita with ¼ cup marinara sauce.

3. Top each pita with chicken, artichokes, and goat cheese.

4. Place in the oven and bake until the cheese is melted, 5 to 6 minutes.

5. Remove from the oven. Cut each pizza into fourths and serve each person two pieces.

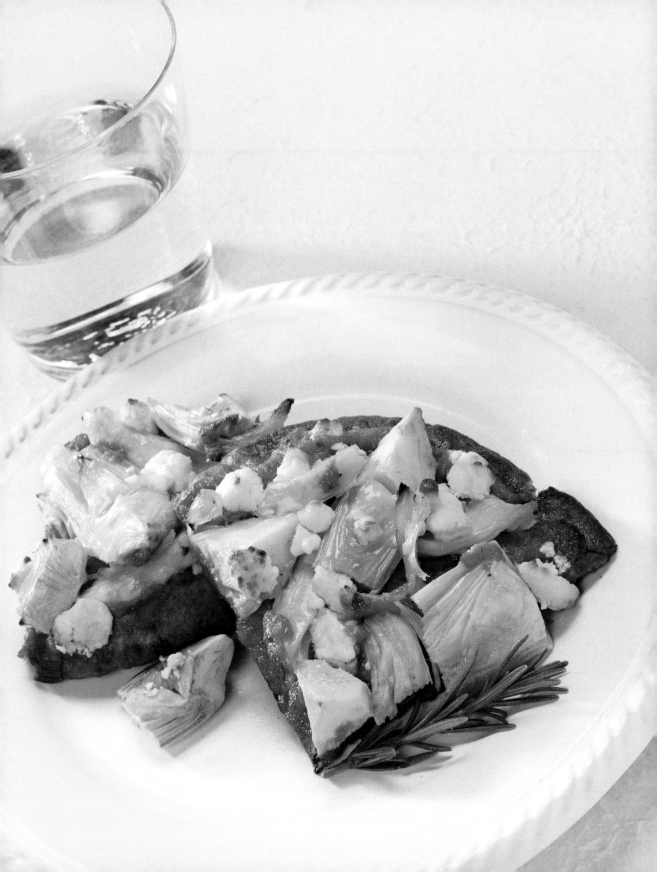

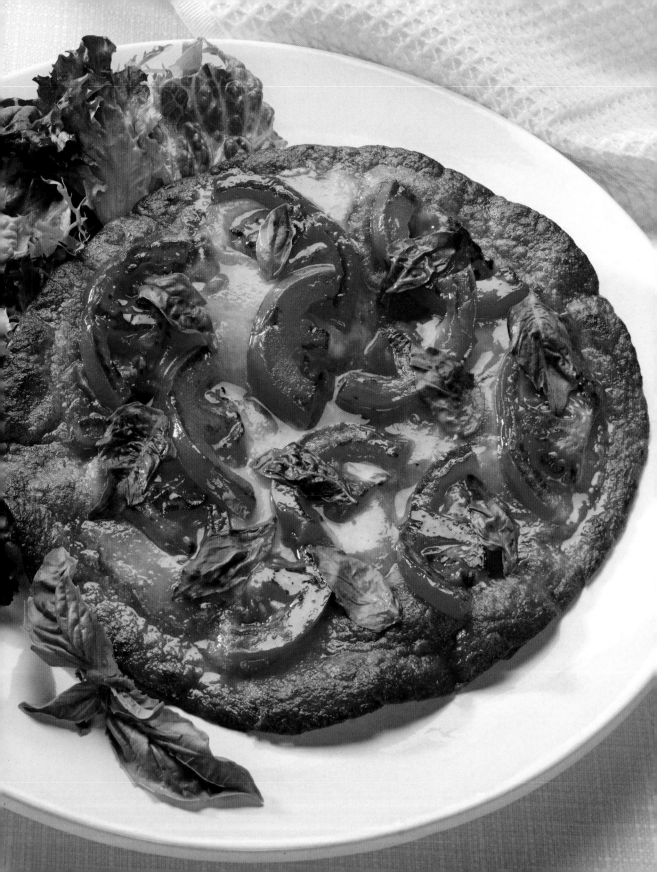

FRESH TOMATO AND MOZZARELLA PIZZA

Italians call this classic pizza "pizza margherita." Fresh, ripe ingredients—garden-fresh summer tomatoes, bright floral basil, and water-packed fresh mozzarella—are key to making this pizza truly savory.

MAKES 4 SERVINGS

Four 6-inch flour tortillas
1 tablespoon olive oil
1 teaspoon garlic powder
12 ounces fresh mozzarella cheese, sliced
2 plum tomatoes, sliced
2 tablespoons chopped fresh basil leaves
Juice of ½ lemon
4 cups mixed salad greens

1. Preheat the oven to 350°F. Line a baking sheet with aluminum foil.

2. Place the tortillas on the baking sheet and drizzle each one with oil. Sprinkle with garlic powder and top with the mozzarella cheese, tomatoes, and basil.

3. Bake until the cheese just melts, 6 to 8 minutes.

4. In a large bowl, squeeze the lemon juice over the salad greens and toss to coat.

5. Carefully remove the tortillas from the oven and serve each person one pizza and one-fourth of the salad.

BLUE CHEESE, RED ONION, AND OLIVE PIZZA

This pizza was created for people who like big flavors. The combination of pungent blue cheese, sharp red onion, and briny olives creates a pizza that's so dense in flavor, no one will know that it's so low in calories.

MAKES 4 SERVINGS

Four 6-inch flour tortillas
4 ounces blue cheese, crumbled, about ½ cup
8 ounces part-skim mozzarella cheese, sliced
½ small red onion, thinly sliced
½ cup chopped olives
4 small pears

1.   Preheat the oven to 350°F. Line a baking sheet with aluminum foil.

2.   Place the tortillas on a baking sheet, top with the cheeses, onion, and olives.

3.   Bake the pizzas until the cheese melts and the tortillas are crisp, 6 to 8 minutes.

4.   Serve each person one pizza and one pear.

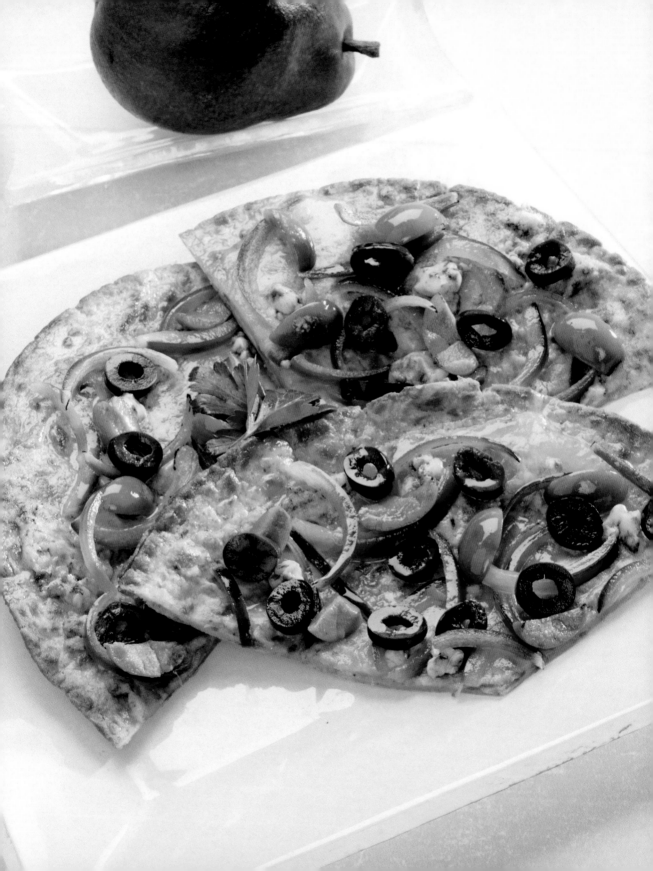

PINEAPPLE RICOTTA PIZZA

Pineapple not only tastes sweet and yummy, but can also aid digestion and reduce inflammation. Pineapple is rich in bromelain, which, in clinical trials, was found to reduce inflammation in sore throats, arthritis, and gout, as well as speeding recovery from surgery and injuries.

MAKES 4 SERVINGS

Four 6-inch flour tortillas
1½ cups skim-milk ricotta cheese
4 ounces sliced pineapple (thawed if frozen, drained if canned)
6 ounces shredded part-skim mozzarella cheese, about ¾ cup
6 ounces cooked chicken breast meat, diced
1 cup cherry tomatoes, halved
4 cups mixed salad greens
½ cup fat-free salad dressing

1. Preheat the oven to 350°F. Line a baking sheet with aluminum foil.

2. Place the tortillas on the baking sheet and top with the ricotta, pineapple, and mozzarella.

3. Bake until the cheese melts and the tortillas are crisp, 6 to 8 minutes.

4. Meanwhile, toss the chicken, tomatoes, and salad greens with the dressing in a large bowl. Divide evenly among four plates.

5. Serve each person one pizza and one salad.

THREE-CHEESE PIZZA

Despite the array of pizza toppings available, cheese remains the most popular. If you're a cheese lover, this pizza won't disappoint you.

MAKES 4 SERVINGS

Four 6-inch flour tortillas
1 cup prepared pizza sauce
4 ounces shredded low-fat cheddar cheese, about ½ cup
4 ounces shredded low-fat Swiss cheese, about ½ cup
4 ounces shredded low-fat mozzarella cheese, about ½ cup
4 cups mixed salad greens
½ cup fat-free salad dressing

1. Preheat the oven to 350°F. Line a baking sheet with aluminum foil.

2. Place the tortillas on the baking sheet and spread with the pizza sauce and top with the cheeses.

3. Bake until the cheese just melts and the tortillas are crisp, 6 to 8 minutes.

4. Meanwhile, toss the salad greens with the dressing in a large bowl and divide equally among four plates.

5. Serve each person one pizza and one salad.

WHITE PIZZA WITH BASIL

This pizza demonstrates how a few simple staple ingredients can create a delicious and satisfying meal in no time. Take a look in your fridge and see how you can dress up this pizza to call the recipe your own.

MAKES 4 SERVINGS

1 tablespoon extra virgin olive oil
Four 6-inch flour tortillas
1 teaspoon garlic powder
1½ cups part-skim ricotta cheese
6 ounces part-skim mozzarella, shredded, about ¾ cup
2 tablespoons chopped basil
4 medium apples

1. Preheat oven to 350°F. Line a baking sheet with aluminum foil.

2. Drizzle the oil on the tortillas and sprinkle with garlic powder. Top with the ricotta, mozzarella, and basil.

3. Bake until the mozzarella melts, 6 to 8 minutes.

4. Serve each person one pizza with one apple.

PIZZA TAPENADE WITH MOZZARELLA

A tapenade is a spread made of, at the very least, black or green olives pureed in olive oil. It can also contain anchovies, capers, garlic, or parsley, and it makes a flavor-packed pizza spread. Tapenade is available in all major supermarkets.

MAKES 4 SERVINGS

Four 6-inch flour tortillas
4 tablespoons prepared black olive tapenade
12 ounces part-skim mozzarella, shredded, about 1½ cups
2 plum tomatoes, sliced thinly
2 scallions, sliced
4 cups mixed salad greens
½ cup fat-free vinaigrette

1. Preheat oven to 350°F. Line a baking sheet with aluminum foil.

2. Place the tortillas on the baking sheet and spread with the tapenade. Top with the mozzarella, tomatoes, and scallions.

3. Bake until the cheese melts, 6 to 8 minutes.

4. Meanwhile, toss the salad greens with vinaigrette in a large bowl.

5. Serve each person one pizza and one salad.

MEDITERRANEAN FRENCH BREAD PIZZA WITH SOUP

Roasted red peppers and crumbled feta cheese add an extra boost of flavor to this unique French bread pizza. Serve it with lentil or bean soup for a satisfying meal.

MAKES 4 SERVINGS

One 12-inch whole grain French baguette
2 cups prepared pizza sauce
2 cups baby spinach
1 jar roasted red peppers, drained and sliced
½ red onion, thinly sliced
4 ounces feta cheese, crumbled, about ½ cup
4 cups Health Valley® Fat Free Black Bean & Vegetable Soup or No Salt Added
    Organic Lentil Soup

1. Preheat the oven to 350°F. Line a baking sheet with aluminum foil.

2. Slice the baguette into two 6-inch pieces and slice each piece in half lengthwise.

3. Toast the bread for 3 to 4 minutes.

4. Spread ¼ cup pizza sauce on top of the toasted bread. Layer with spinach, pepper slices, onion, and feta.

5. Return the baguette to the oven for 4 to 5 minutes more until all the ingredients are hot and the spinach is wilted.

6. While the pizza bakes, heat the soup in a microwave according to the package instructions.

7. Serve each person one pizza with 1 cup of soup.

CHICKEN AND VEGETABLE PIZZA

Sometimes the best lunches are last night's leftovers. This recipe makes two extra pieces of pizza to enjoy the following day.

MAKES 4 SERVINGS

Two 12-inch whole wheat pizza crusts
2 cups prepared pizza sauce
4 ounces part-skim milk mozzarella cheese, shredded, about ½ cup
2 ounces Parmesan, grated, about 2 tablespoons
12 ounces cooked chicken breast meat, diced
1 green bell pepper, sliced
1 cup sliced mushrooms
One 2½-ounce can sliced black olives, drained
4 cups mixed salad greens
¼ cup reduced-fat vinaigrette

1. Preheat the oven to 375°F.

2. Toast the pizza crusts on a rack in oven for 3 to 4 minutes.

3. Carefully remove from the oven and spread with the pizza sauce. Layer with the cheeses, chicken breast, green pepper, mushrooms, and olives.

4. Bake until the cheese is melted, 7 to 10 minutes. Remove from the oven and transfer to a large cutting board. Let the pizza cool while you prepare the salad.

5. Toss salad greens with vinaigrette in a large bowl and divide evenly among four salad plates.

6. Slice each pizza into thirds. Serve each person one-third of a pizza with one salad. Reserve the two remaining pieces of pizza for a later meal.

Chapter 7
FISH & SEAFOOD

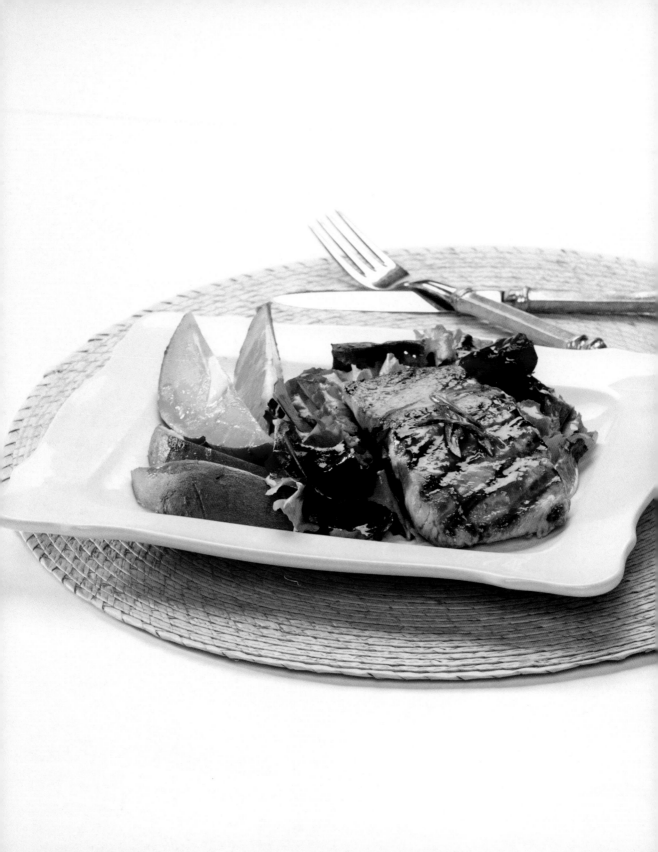

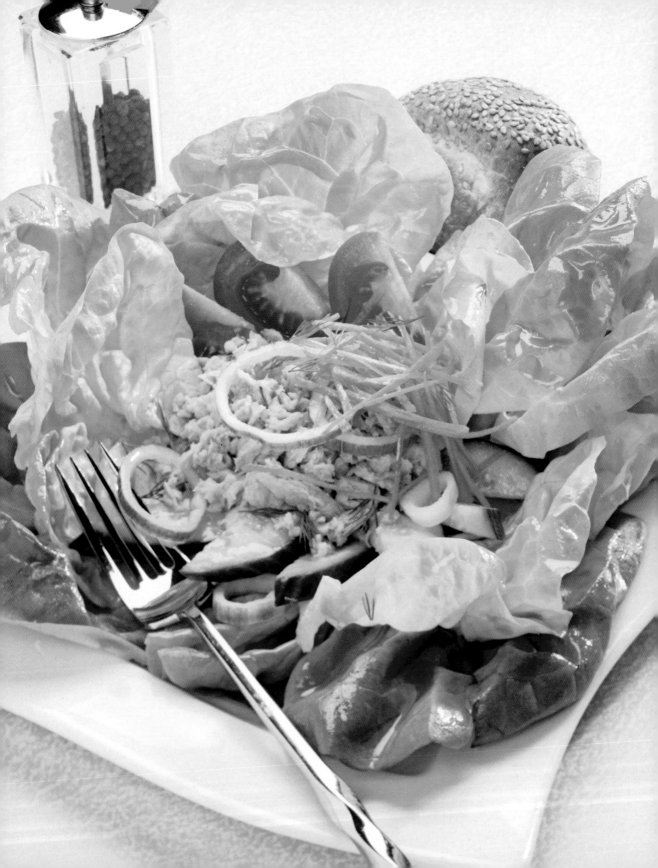

COLD TUNA PLATTER

Tuna is an excellent source of heart-healthy omega-3 fatty acids. If you like, substitute with other omega-3 rich fish, such as salmon, sardines, or mackerel.

MAKES 4 SERVINGS

6 cups shredded Bibb lettuce
Four 3-ounce cans tuna in water, drained
2 tomatoes, sliced
1 red onion, thinly sliced
1 cucumber, sliced
1 cup shredded carrots
4 sprigs dill
4 small whole grain rolls

For the dressing
¼ cup red wine vinegar
1 teaspoon dried Italian seasoning
1 teaspoon garlic powder
2 teaspoons sugar
4 teaspoons extra virgin olive oil

1. Arrange 1½ cups Bibb lettuce on each of four plates.

2. Empty one can of tuna on each plate.

3. Garnish each plate evenly with the tomatoes, onion, cucumber, and carrots.

4. Place a sprig of dill on top of the tuna.

5. Whisk together the red wine vinegar, Italian seasoning, sugar, and garlic powder in a small bowl. Slowly stream in the olive oil, whisking constantly. Drizzle the dressing over the salads.

6. Serve each person one salad with a whole grain roll.

GRILLED SHRIMP, HUMMUS, AND VEGGIE PLATTER

Hummus makes a delicious alternative to sour cream-based vegetable dips. Although not necessarily lower in fat, hummus provides heart-healthy unsaturated fat as well as considerable protein to a fresh vegetable platter.

MAKES 4 SERVINGS

Cooking spray
1 tablespoon olive oil
1 teaspoon salt
2 teaspoons garlic powder
2 zucchini, sliced lengthwise into ¼-inch planks
1 red or yellow onion, sliced into 2-inch-thick pieces, rings kept intact
6 cups mixed salad greens
1 cup hummus
8 ounces cooked shrimp, thawed if frozen
½ cup sliced roasted red peppers (jarred)
20 olives
1 cup cherry tomatoes
1 cup carrots, cut into matchsticks
1 cucumber, peeled and sliced

For the dressing
6 tablespoons low-fat Italian dressing
¼ cup plain nonfat yogurt
2 tablespoons pre-minced garlic
2 tablespoons lemon juice, about 1 lemon
2 whole grain pita breads, halved

1. Preheat a grill or grill pan to medium and spray with cooking spray.

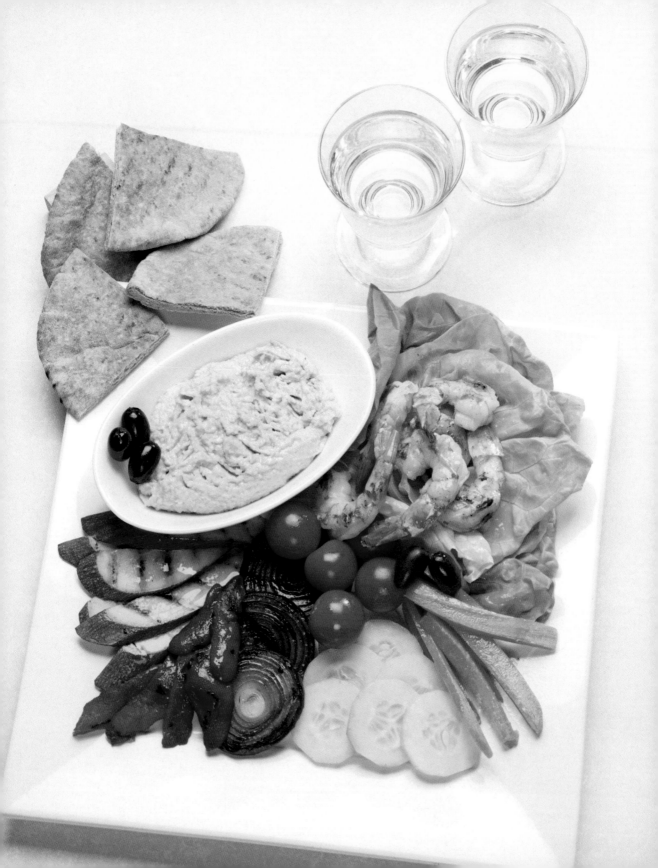

2.   Whisk together the olive oil, salt, and garlic powder in a small bowl. Add the zucchini and onion and toss to coat.

3.   Grill the zucchini and onion until they soften and turn golden brown, 3 to 4 minutes per side.

4.   On each of four plates, arrange 1½ cups mixed salad greens, ¼ cup hummus, 2 ounces shrimp, 2 tablespoons peppers, 5 olives, ¼ cup cherry tomatoes, ¼ cup carrots, and one-fourth of the cucumber.

5.   Stir together the Italian dressing, yogurt, garlic, and lemon juice in a small bowl and pour evenly over the salad.

6.   Serve each person one salad with half a pita bread.

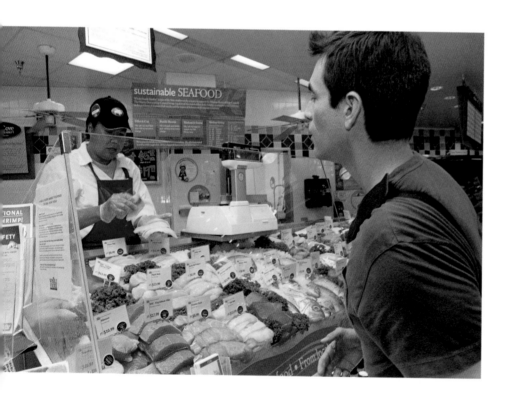

QUICK-BROILED FLOUNDER

Flounder is a flatfish that's affordable and widely available. The thin fillets are well-suited to quick-cooking; they cook so quickly, there's no need to turn them while broiling.

MAKES 4 SERVINGS

2 medium sweet potatoes, cut in half lengthwise
One 10-ounce box frozen mixed vegetables
Cooking spray
Four 4-ounce flounder fillets
4 teaspoons butter, melted
1 teaspoon seasoned salt, such as Lawry's®
2 tablespoons garlic powder
1 tablespoon lemon juice, about ½ lemon
¼ cup white wine
Lemon wedges

1. Preheat the broiler.

2. Pierce the sweet potatoes and microwave on high for 6 to 7 minutes until tender.

3. Cook the vegetables according to the package instructions.

4. Spray a baking sheet with cooking spray.

5. Place the flounder on the baking sheet. Brush the fillets with butter and sprinkle with seasoned salt, garlic powder, lemon juice, and white wine.

6. Broil the fillets until the fish flakes easily with a fork, 5 minutes, taking care not to overcook.

7. Serve each person one fillet with lemon wedges, half a sweet potato, and ½ cup of vegetables.

COLD SHRIMP PLATTER WITH MANGO, ONION, TOMATO, AND CHICKPEAS

This platter makes a perfect light summer lunch. For best results, choose ripe, summer-fresh mangoes and tomatoes that are at their peak of flavor.

MAKES 4 SERVINGS

6 cups mixed salad greens
10 ounces cooked shrimp (thawed if frozen)
1 cup chickpeas, rinsed and drained
1 mango, sliced
1 red onion, sliced
1 cup cherry tomatoes
4 tablespoons low-fat Italian dressing
2 whole grain pita breads, halved

1. Combine the greens, shrimp, chickpeas, mango, onion, and tomatoes in a large bowl. Add the dressing and toss to coat.

2. Divide the salad equally among four plates.

3. Serve each person one salad with half a pita bread.

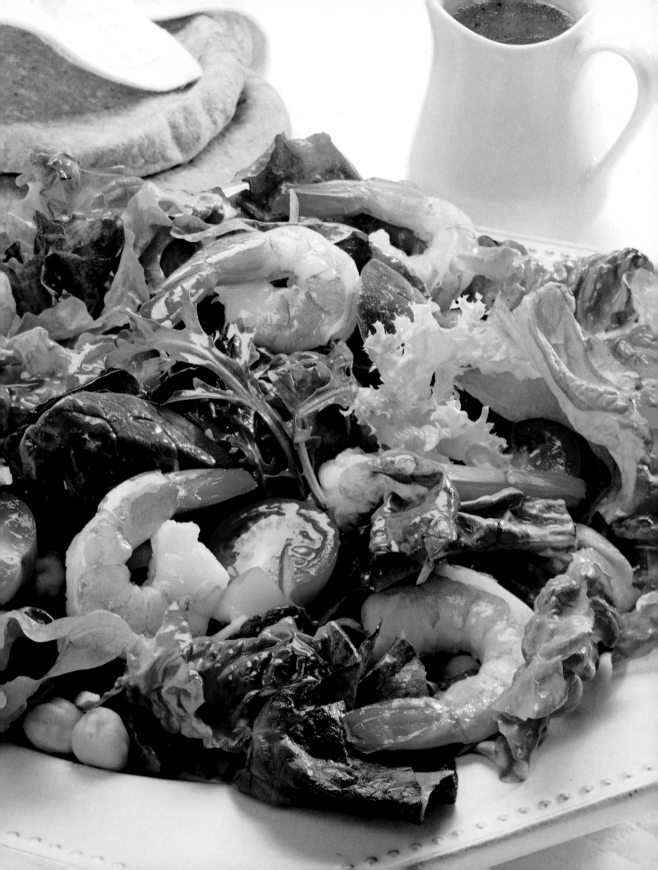

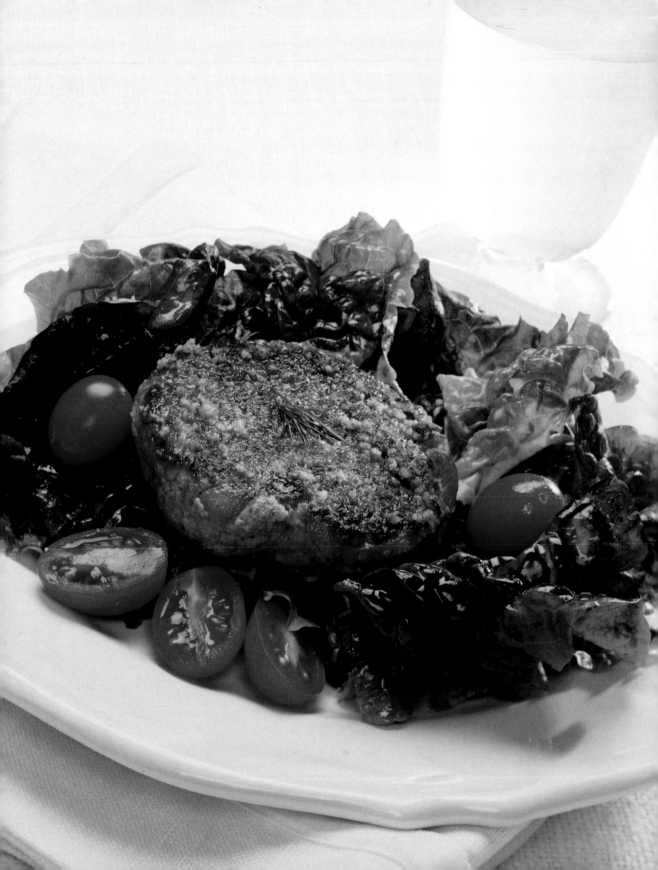

SALMON CAKES

Salmon is one of the healthiest foods you can eat. Not only is it chockfull of omega-3 fatty acids, which promote heart health, but salmon is also an excellent source of low-fat protein, niacin, vitamin B_{12}, phosphorous, magnesium, and vitamin B_6.

MAKES 4 SERVINGS

One 6-ounce pouch or can water-packed salmon
1 tablespoon grill seasoning, such as McCormick's Grill Mates®
¼ cup low-fat mayonnaise
1 tablespoon lemon juice, about ½ lemon
1 egg, lightly beaten
¾ cup plain dried bread crumbs
Cooking spray
1 tablespoon olive oil
4 cups mixed salad greens
1 pint grape tomatoes, cut in half
¼ cup fat-free balsamic vinaigrette

1. Gently fold the salmon, grill seasoning, mayonnaise, lemon juice, egg, and bread crumbs together, taking care not to break up the salmon flakes too much.

2. Shape salmon mixture into four equal patties.

3. Heat a large nonstick skillet over medium heat, spray with cooking spray, and add oil.

4. Add salmon cakes to skillet and cook 2 to 3 minutes on each side until browned.

5. Meanwhile, combine the salad greens and tomatoes in a large bowl and toss with the dressing. Divide the salad evenly among four plates.

6. Serve each person one salmon patty with one salad.

QUICK FISH TACOS

This savory, one-dish meal is a healthy, quick, and easy foray into the flavors of Mexico.

MAKES 4 SERVINGS

Cooking spray
One 10-ounce package frozen, cooked, unbreaded fish fillets
½ packet taco seasoning
One 12-ounce package broccoli slaw
1 tablespoon extra virgin olive oil
8 hard corn taco shells
2 tomatoes, chopped
6 ounces shredded Mexican cheese blend

1. Preheat the oven to 400°F.

2. Spray a baking dish with cooking spray and add the fish.

3. Sprinkle the fish with 1 tablespoon of the taco seasoning and bake until the fish flakes easily with a fork, 6 to 7 minutes.

4. Meanwhile, toss the broccoli slaw with the oil and remaining taco seasoning in a large bowl.

5. Place ½ cup broccoli slaw in each taco shell. Break the fish into bite-size pieces and divide evenly among taco shells. Top with the tomatoes and cheese.

6. Serve each person two tacos.

CHEESY SALMON QUESADILLAS

This recipe demonstrates how versatile this Mexican sandwich can be. Experiment with various cheeses, meat, fish, and vegetables to create a quesadilla that's uniquely yours.

MAKES 4 SERVINGS

Cooking spray
One 6-ounce pouch or can water-packed salmon
4 ounces shredded Monterey Jack cheese, about ½ cup
One 8-ounce jar roasted red peppers, drained and sliced
2 green onions, sliced
Four 6-inch flour tortillas
1 avocado, pitted and sliced into 4 pieces
1 cup salsa
¼ cup chopped cilantro

1. Heat a large nonstick skillet over medium heat and spray with cooking spray.

2. Divide the salmon, cheese, peppers, and green onions among two tortillas. Top with remaining two tortillas.

3. Put the quesadillas in the heated pan, one at a time, and cook, flipping once, until the cheese is melted and the tortillas are golden brown on both sides, 4 to 5 minutes per side. Remove to a large cutting board and slice into fourths.

4. Serve each person half a quesadilla garnished with one slice of avocado, ¼ cup salsa, and 1 tablespoon cilantro.

BARBECUED SALMON

Take pleasure in barbecued salmon and sweet potatoes and know that in addition to protein and complex carbs, your family is getting rich dietary fiber, vitamins A and C, and a health dose of vitamin B_6.

MAKES 4 SERVINGS

Four 4-ounce salmon fillets
6 tablespoons prepared barbecue sauce
4 small sweet potatoes
4 cups mixed salad greens
4 tablespoons fat-free Italian dressing
2 green onions, sliced
4 teaspoons butter or Better Butter (see page 23)

1. Preheat a grill pan or George Foreman–type grill to medium.

2. Brush salmon with barbecue sauce and grill until it flakes easily with a fork, 3 to 4 minutes per side, turning once if in a grill pan.

3. Meanwhile, pierce sweet potatoes with a fork and microwave on high until tender, 3 to 4 minutes per side.

4. In a large bowl, toss the salad greens with the dressing. Divide evenly among four plates.

5. Serve each person one piece of salmon garnished with green onions, one sweet potato, sliced and topped with butter, and one salad.

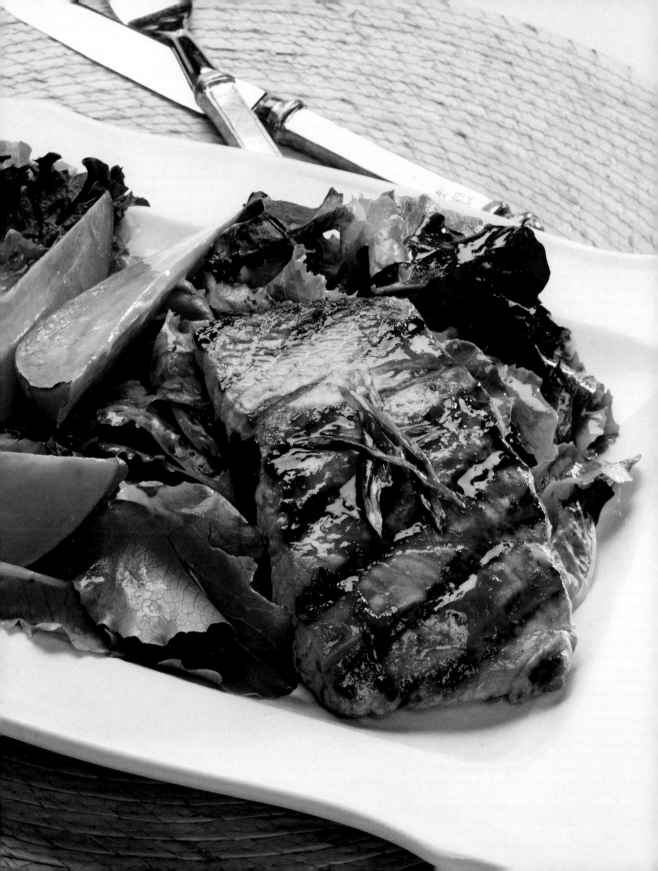

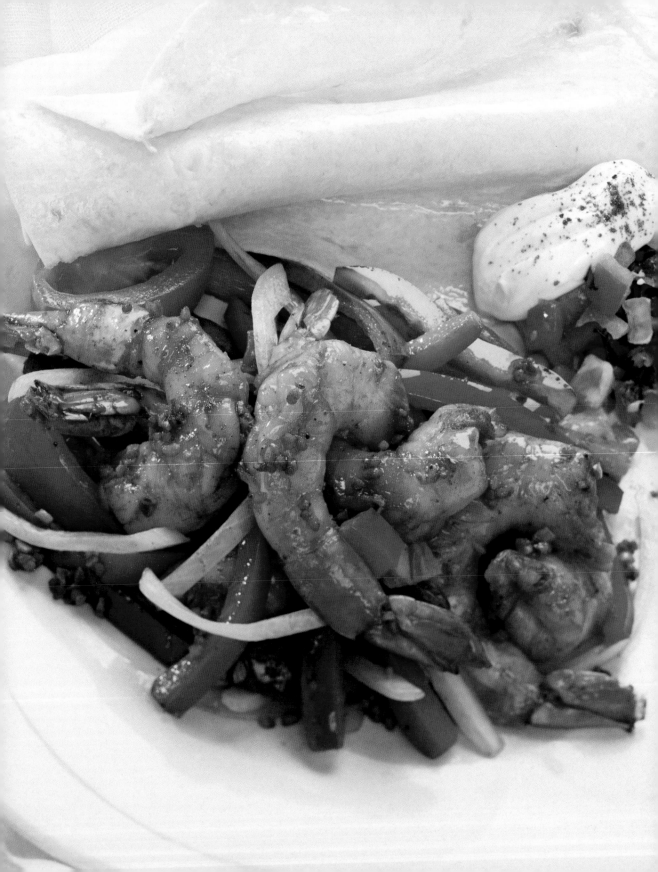

SHRIMP FAJITA STIR-FRY

Stir-frying is a valuable technique to learn because very little oil is necessary and the food cooks very quickly. To save even more time, buy precut stir-fry vegetables; they're sold near the bagged salad mixes in most supermarkets.

Makes 4 servings

4 teaspoons canola oil
2 red bell peppers, cut into strips
1 green bell pepper, cut into strips
1 large onion, sliced
2 tomatoes, cut into wedges
2 tablespoons minced garlic
1 teaspoon freshly ground black pepper
1 teaspoon salt
2 teaspoons paprika
2 tablespoons low-sodium soy sauce
2 tablespoons lime juice, about 2 limes
12 ounces cooked shrimp (thawed if frozen)
Four 6-inch flour tortillas
¼ cup nonfat sour cream
½ cup prepared salsa

1. Heat a wok or large skillet over high heat and add the oil.

2. Add the bell peppers, onion, and tomatoes to the wok and stir-fry until tender, 5 minutes.

3. Stir together the garlic, pepper, salt, paprika, soy sauce, and lime juice in a small bowl, and then add to the wok, stirring to coat the vegetables in the sauce.

4. Add the shrimp and cook until heated through, 1 to 2 minutes.

5. Divide the shrimp mixture equally among four plates and serve with one tortilla, 1 tablespoon sour cream, and 2 tablespoons salsa.

SAUTÉED SCALLOPS WITH SPINACH OVER POLENTA

Sweet, tiny bay scallops are perfect for quick-cooking meals. Look for pale beige to creamy pink scallops; if they're bright white, they've been soaked in water and therefore won't brown as well.

MAKES 4 SERVINGS

Cooking spray
Eight ½-inch slices prepared polenta
1 ounce grated Parmesan, about 1 tablespoon
1 tablespoon olive oil
2 tablespoons minced garlic
¾ pound bay scallops
½ teaspoon salt
¼ teaspoon white pepper
1 tablespoon lemon juice, about ½ lemon
½ cup low-sodium chicken broth
2 tablespoons dried minced onion
1 package baby spinach

1. Preheat the oven to 400°F. Spray a baking sheet with cooking spray.

2. Place the polenta slices on baking sheet and top with Parmesan. Bake until the polenta develops a golden crust, 6 to 8 minutes.

3. Meanwhile, heat a large nonstick skillet over medium-high heat and add the oil, garlic, and scallops. Cook for 2 minutes.

4. Turn the scallops and cook for 1 to 2 minutes more. Add the lemon juice, chicken broth, onion, and spinach. Cover and cook until the spinach is wilted, 1 to 2 minutes.

5. Place two slices of polenta on each of four plates. Divide the scallop mixture evenly over the polenta and serve.

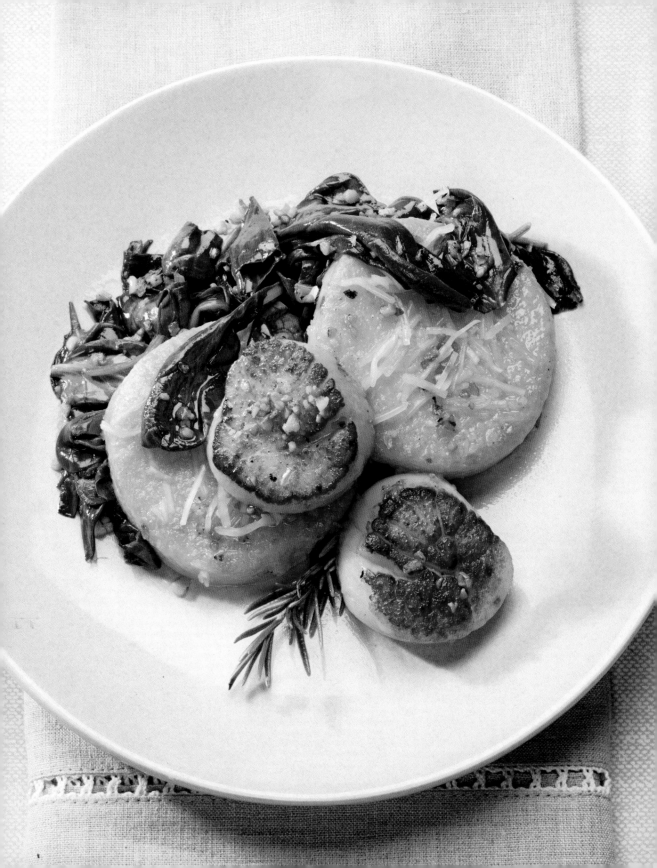

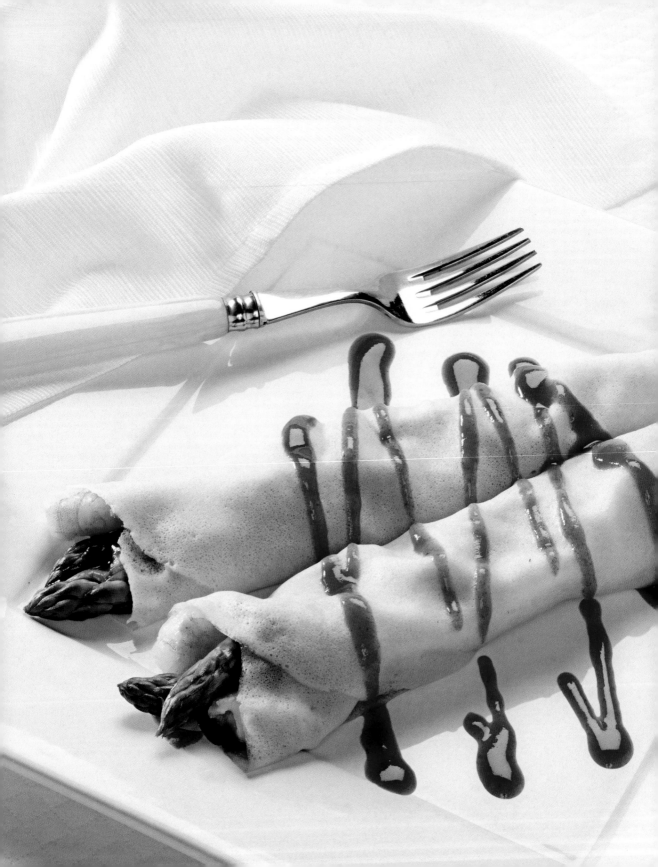

SHRIMP AND ASPARAGUS CREPES

If you like asparagus, you'll love these crepes. Buy prepared crepes and this extraordinary meal will be ready to eat in minutes.

MAKES 4 SERVINGS

1 pound asparagus spears
Cooking spray
1 pound uncooked shrimp, cleaned and deveined
Salt and freshly ground black pepper
½ cup prepared barbecue sauce
Eight 9-inch prepared crepes

1. Place the asparagus in a microwave-safe dish with 2 tablespoons of water and microwave until tender, 5 to 6 minutes. Set aside.

2. Meanwhile, heat a large nonstick skillet over medium-high heat and spray with cooking spray.

3. Season the shrimp with salt and pepper and add to skillet.

4. Cook the shrimp for 1 to 2 minutes per side (turning once) or until nearly opaque. Stir in the barbecue sauce and reduce heat to low. Bring the sauce to a simmer.

5. Warm the crepes in the microwave for 30 seconds.

6. Divide the shrimp mixture evenly among the crepes. Top with asparagus. Roll the crepes into a cigar shape.

7. Serve each person two crepes.

BROILED SALMON AND BRUSSELS SPROUTS

When prepared correctly, Brussels sprouts are crispy little cabbages that not only look pretty and taste delicious, but also contain phytochemicals that help protect the body from several diseases, including cancer.

MAKES 4 SERVINGS

8 ounces soba noodles
Cooking spray
Four 4-ounce skinless salmon fillets
1½ pounds Brussels sprouts, trimmed and halved lengthwise
2 tablespoons safflower or canola oil
½ teaspoon coarse salt
¼ teaspoon freshly ground black pepper
2 teaspoons toasted sesame oil
2 teaspoons toasted sesame seeds
2 tablespoons chopped chives

1. Cook the soba noodles according to the package instructions.

2. Preheat the broiler. Spray a baking sheet with cooking spray.

3. Place the salmon fillets on the baking sheet and surround with the Brussels sprouts.

4. Drizzle the oil over the Brussels sprouts and salmon and season with salt and pepper.

5. Broil until the salmon is cooked to desired doneness, 7 minutes for medium.

6. Drain the soba noodles and toss with the sesame oil and sesame seeds.

7. Serve each person one salmon fillet, one-fourth of the Brussels sprouts, and one-fourth of the sesame soba noodles. Garnish the plates with chopped chives.

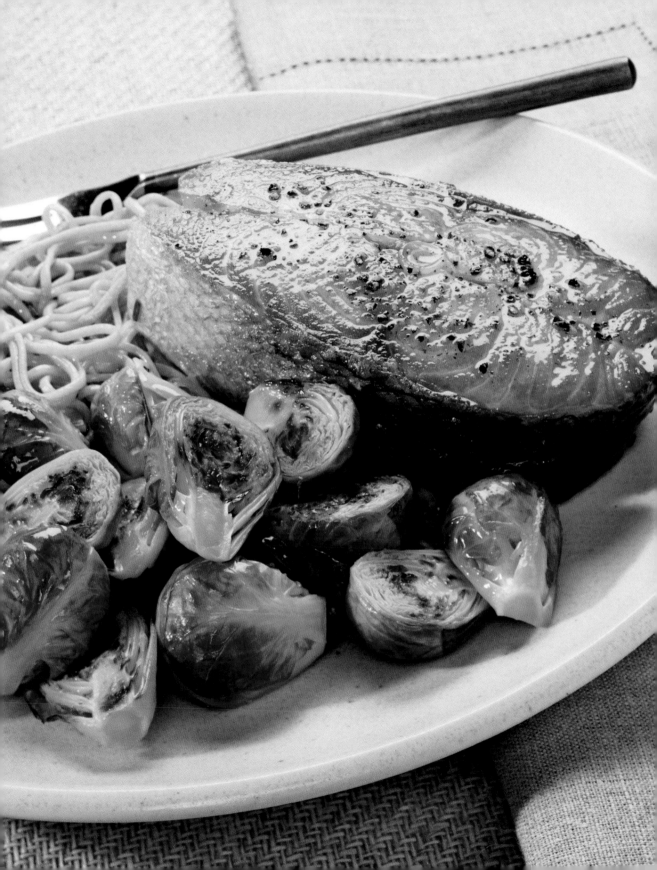

GRILLED TILAPIA

Tilapia is a firm-fleshed white fish that's well-suited to baking, broiling, grilling, and steaming. In this recipe, we pair tilapia with grilled polenta, or Italian cornmeal mush, and crisp green beans.

MAKES 4 SERVINGS

Cooking spray
2 cups frozen whole green beans
Four 4-ounce tilapia fillets
Four 1-inch slices prepared polenta
2 tablespoons extra virgin olive oil
2 teaspoons seasoned salt, such as Lawry's®

1. Heat a George Foreman–type grill to medium and spray with cooking spray.

2. Combine the green beans with 2 tablespoons water in a medium microwave-safe dish. Microwave until heated through, 3 minutes.

3. Brush the fish and polenta with the olive oil and sprinkle with seasoned salt.

4. Place the fish and polenta on the grill and cook 3 to 4 minutes on each side, turning once, until the fish flakes easily with a fork and the polenta develops a crisp, brown crust.

5. Serve each person one fish fillet with one slice of polenta and ½ cup of green beans.

SALMON AND BROWN RICE

This meal demonstrates how even a simple combination can make a substantial, flavorful, healthy dinner. Butterfly your fillets to make them thinner, about a half inch thick, which will help them cook much faster.

MAKES 4 SERVINGS

1 cup quick-cooking brown rice
Cooking spray
Four 4-ounce salmon fillets
2 tablespoons lemon juice, about 1 lemon
2 tablespoons chopped dill
Salt and freshly ground black pepper
One 10-ounce bag mixed vegetables (frozen can substitute for fresh)
1 tablespoon extra virgin olive oil

1. Preheat the oven to 375°F.

2. Combine the rice with 2 cups water in a medium saucepan over medium heat and cover. Bring to a boil and reduce heat to low. Simmer until the rice is tender and has absorbed all the water, about 10 minutes.

3. Spray a baking sheet with cooking spray.

4. Slice the salmon fillets widthwise without cutting all the way through, and open them like a book. Place on the baking sheet.

5. Pour the lemon juice over the salmon and sprinkle with the dill, salt, and pepper. Bake the salmon to desired doneness, 7 minutes for medium.

6. While the fish bakes, bring about 2 inches of water to a simmer in a large stockpot and add a steamer basket. Add the vegetables and cover. Steam the vegetables until tender, 6 minutes.

7. Remove the vegetables to a large bowl and toss with the oil and a pinch of salt.

8. Serve each person one piece of salmon with ½ cup of rice and one-fourth of the vegetables.

CAJUN CATFISH WITH SAUTÉED GREENS

Cajun seasonings vary from brand to brand. If you like, you can make your own; most Cajun rubs include dried thyme, paprika, dry mustard, garlic powder, cayenne pepper, dried sage, and salt. Experiment with different quantities of these ingredients and add others until you create a seasoning that you can call your own.

MAKES 4 SERVINGS

Four 4-ounce skinless catfish fillets
1½ tablespoons Cajun seasoning
1 tablespoon olive oil
2 sweet potatoes
1 teaspoon minced garlic
2 bunches or 1 large bag of braising greens, such as chard, collards, or mustard greens, sliced into ribbons
½ teaspoon balsamic vinegar
Salt to taste

1. Preheat the broiler.

2. Place the catfish fillets in an oven-safe dish large enough to hold them in one layer and sprinkle with the Cajun seasoning.

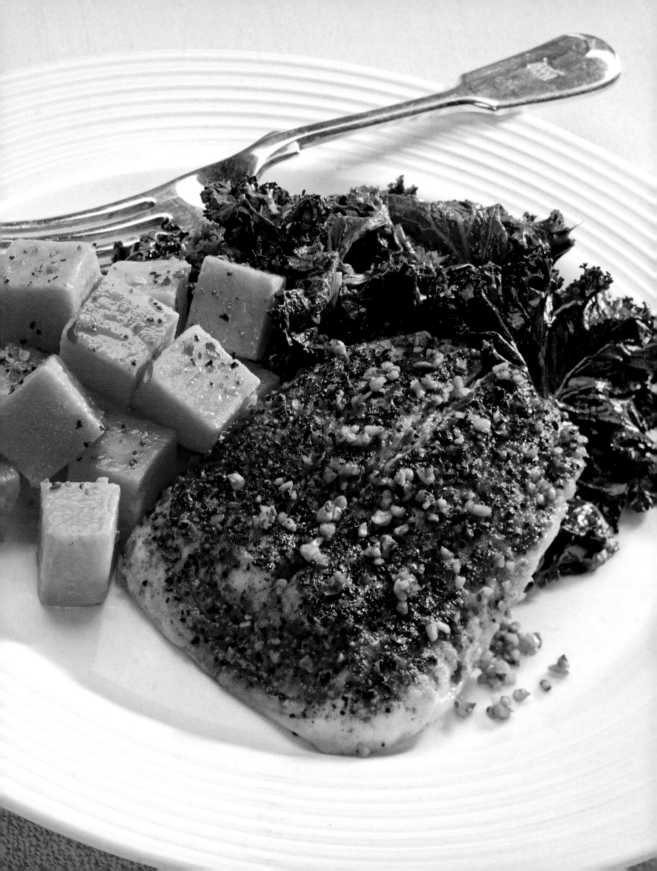

3.   Broil the fish for 5 minutes, flip, and broil until fish is opaque and flakes easily with a fork, 5 minutes more.

4.   While the fish broils, pierce the sweet potatoes with a fork and microwave on high for 3 to 4 minutes and turn. Microwave for another 3 to 4 minutes until tender. Remove from the microwave and slice in half lengthwise.

5.   Heat a large skillet over medium heat and add the oil.

6.   Add the garlic to the skillet and sauté until golden, 30 seconds. Add the greens and cook until wilted, 5 minutes. Remove from heat and stir in the vinegar and salt to taste.

7.   Serve each person one piece of fish with half a sweet potato and one-fourth of the greens.

CHILI LIME SHRIMP WITH BROWN RICE AND TOASTED PECANS

Sweet, smoky, spicy chili powder pairs well with tart lime juice to season grilled shrimp in this recipe. Accompanied by nutty brown rice and refreshing fruit, this meal is as delicious as it is beautiful.

MAKES 4 SERVINGS

1 cup quick-cooking brown rice
2 cups vegetable broth
1 tablespoon dried minced onion
2 tablespoons lime juice, about 2 limes
2 teaspoons extra virgin olive oil
¾ teaspoon chili powder

¾ pound uncooked shrimp, shelled and deveined
2 tablespoons chopped pecans
1 green onion, sliced
2 cups mixed fruit salad (thawed if frozen, drained if canned)

1. Heat a grill pan or George Foreman–type grill to medium. Preheat oven to 400°F.

2. Combine the rice, broth, and onion in a medium saucepan over medium heat and cover. Bring to a boil and reduce heat to low. Simmer until the rice is tender and has absorbed all the broth, 10 minutes.

3. Mix 1 tablespoon lime juice, oil, and ½ teaspoon chili powder in a small bowl. Brush over the shrimp. Marinate the shrimp on the countertop while preparing the pecans.

4. Spread the pecans on a baking sheet. Sprinkle with the remaining chili powder. Toast in the oven for 4 to 5 minutes or until fragrant.

5. Place the shrimp on the grill and cook for 2 to 3 minutes per side until opaque, turning once.

6. While the shrimp grills, toss the fruit with the remaining lime juice. Divide equally into four portions.

7. Divide the rice evenly among four plates. Top the rice with shrimp and sprinkle with pecans and green onion. Serve with the fruit.

WHITE FISH AND POTATOES

Breaded and baked white fish eliminates the fat but maintains the flavor of a Midwestern family favorite: fried fish. Served with potatoes and spinach, this meal is as comforting as it is delicious.

MAKES 4 SERVINGS

Cooking spray
¼ cup seasoned bread crumbs
1 pound white fish, such as perch, cod, or orange roughy
1 tablespoon lemon juice, about ½ lemon
4 red potatoes
3 cups bagged baby spinach
2 tablespoons extra virgin olive oil
Pinch of salt

1. Preheat the oven to 375°F. Spray a baking sheet with cooking spray.

2. Place the bread crumbs and fish fillets into a large plastic zip-top bag and shake until the fish is coated.

3. Place the fish on the baking sheet and bake until cooked through, 10 minutes. Pour the lemon juice over the fish.

4. While the fish bakes, pierce the potatoes with a fork and microwave 3 to 4 minutes and turn. Microwave another 3 to 4 minutes until tender.

5. Bring 2 inches of water to a simmer in a large stockpot and add a steamer basket. Add the spinach to the steamer basket, cover, and steam until tender, 1 minute. Drizzle olive oil over the spinach and season with salt.

6. Serve each person one piece of fish, one potato, and one-fourth of the spinach.

AHI TERIYAKI

Ahi is the Hawaiian name for yellowfin tuna. Tuna is an excellent source of low-fat protein as well as omega-3 fatty acids, B vitamins, and essential minerals, including selenium, magnesium, and potassium. Look for bright, glistening tuna steaks that are deep red in color.

MAKES 4 SERVINGS

¼ cup teriyaki sauce
1 tablespoon dry sherry
1 teaspoon grated ginger
2 teaspoons garlic powder
Four 4-ounce ahi steaks
1 cup quick-cooking rice
4 teaspoons extra virgin olive oil
Cooking spray
2 cups mixed fruit salad (thawed if frozen, drained if canned)

1. Stir together the teriyaki sauce, sherry, ginger, and garlic powder in a dish large enough to hold all of the ahi steaks.

2. Add the fish to the marinade, turning to coat. Set aside to marinate.

3. Combine the rice with 2 cups water in a medium saucepan over medium heat and cover. Bring to a boil and reduce heat to low. Simmer until the rice is tender and has absorbed all the water, 10 minutes. Toss the rice with the oil.

4. Heat a large, heavy-bottomed nonstick skillet over high heat until very hot and spray with cooking spray.

5. Remove the tuna from the marinade and pat dry.

6. Sear the tuna for 1 minute per side, working in batches if pieces of the fish don't fit in the skillet. Cook longer if desired, but ahi steaks should be served rare for best flavor.

7. Serve each person one tuna steak, ½ cup of rice, and ½ cup of fruit salad.

Chapter 8
POULTRY

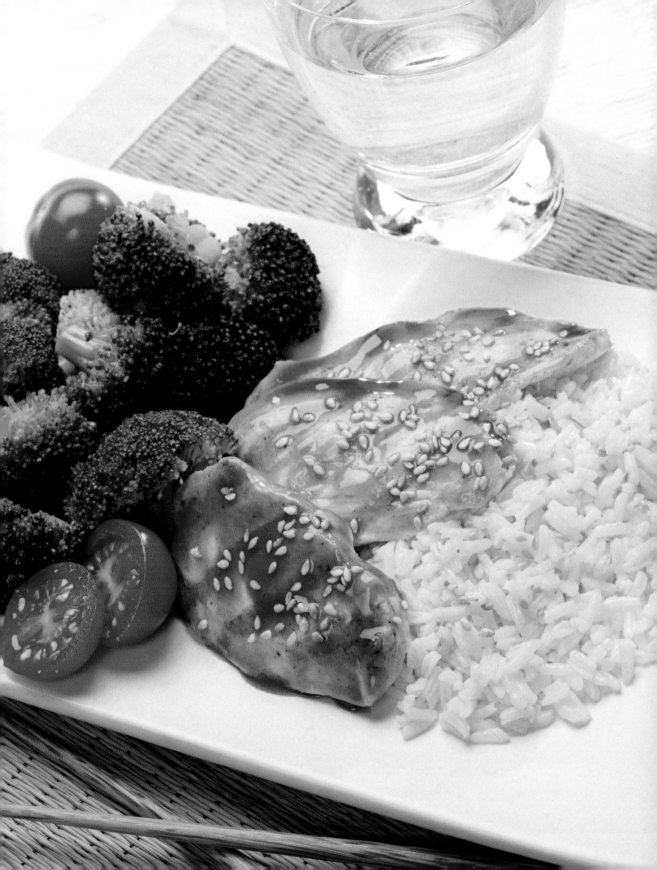

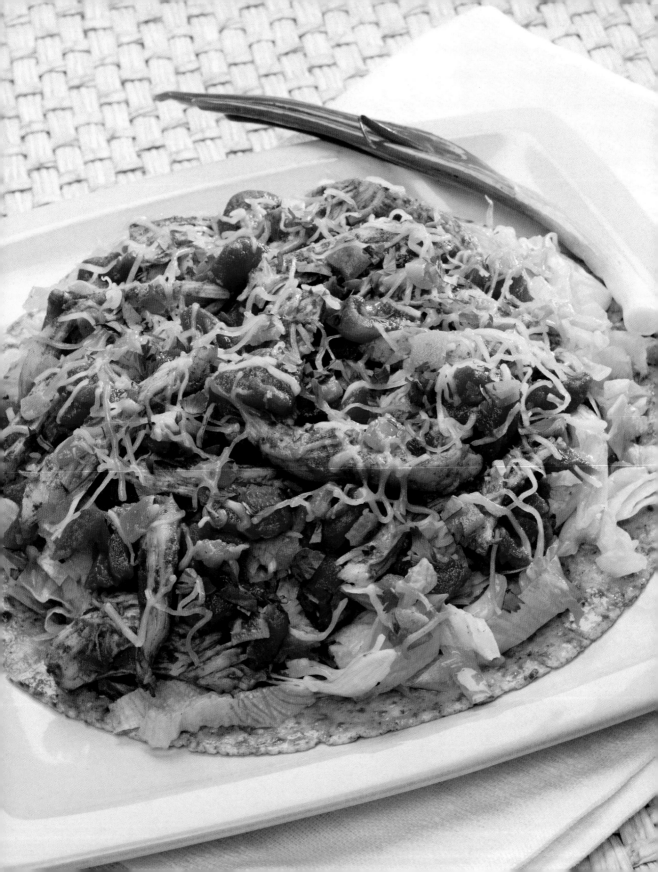

CHICKEN AND CHEESE TOSTADAS

Using baked tortillas instead of fried, low-fat cheese, and chicken breast meat lightens the calorie load of traditional tostadas, so you can still enjoy your favorite south-of-the-border dish.

MAKES 4 SERVINGS

Cooking spray
Four 10-inch flour tortillas
One 1¼ ounce-package dry fajita seasoning mix
4 green onions
6 ounces cooked chicken breast meat, diced
One 15-ounce can diced tomatoes with peppers and onions
¾ cup shredded low-fat Mexican cheese blend
2 cups mixed salad greens
1 tablespoon chopped fresh cilantro or 2 teaspoons dried cilantro

1. Preheat the oven to 400°F. Heat a grill or grill pan to medium-high and spray with cooking spray. Line a baking sheet with aluminum foil.

2. Spray the tortillas with cooking spray and place on baking sheet. Sprinkle with 1 teaspoon the seasoning mix. Bake until crisp, 6 to 7 minutes.

3. Add the green onions to the grill and cook, turning frequently, until softened and lightly browned, 3 minutes. Set aside.

4. Heat a large skillet over medium heat. Add the chicken, the remaining seasoning mix, and the tomatoes to the skillet. Bring the mixture to a boil and reduce heat to low. Simmer for 5 minutes.

5. Remove from heat and stir in ½ cup of the cheese.

6. Place one tortilla on each of four plates. Top with salad greens and the chicken mixture. Sprinkle with the remaining cheese and the cilantro. Serve each person one tostada with a grilled green onion.

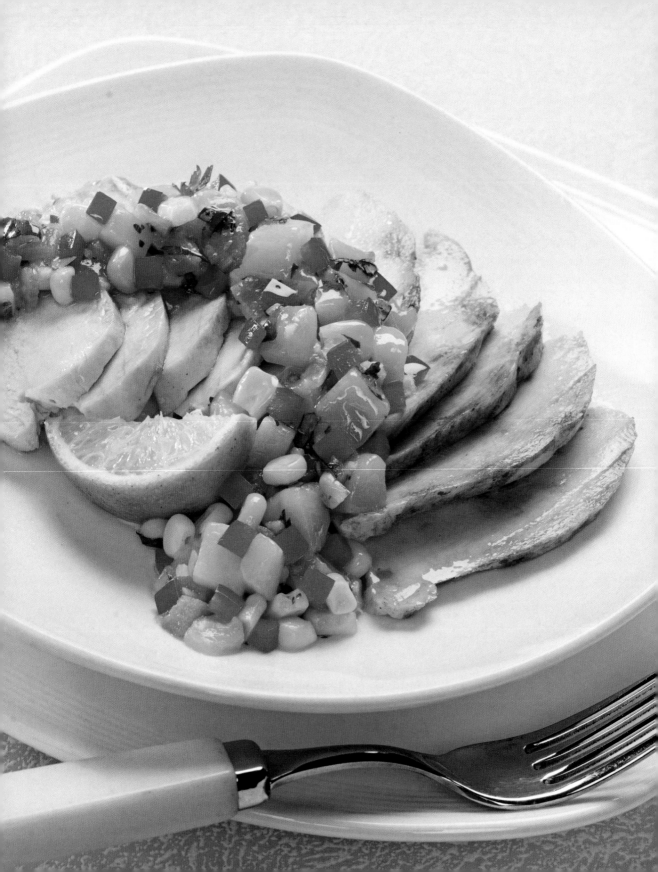

GRILLED CHICKEN WITH MANGO CORN SALSA

Fresh mango salsa is easy to make and delicious served over halibut, salmon, or chicken. Feel free to make a large batch of the salsa, knowing that it will stay fresh a few days.

MAKES 4 SERVINGS

1 pound boneless, skinless chicken breast tenders
1 tablespoon olive oil
½ teaspoon seasoned salt, such as Lawry's®
2 cups diced mango (jarred or frozen can substitute for fresh)
2 cups frozen corn, thawed
2 tablespoons lime juice, about 2 limes
One 4½-ounce can chopped green chiles, drained
1 tablespoon minced garlic
1 teaspoon dried cilantro

1. Heat a grill pan or George Foreman–type grill to medium-high.

2. Brush the chicken with the oil and sprinkle with seasoned salt. Place on the grill and cook for 2 to 3 minutes and turn. Cook for another 2 to 3 minutes until no pink remains.

3. Meanwhile, mix the diced mango with corn, lime juice to taste, chiles, garlic, and cilantro in a small bowl.

4. Place one-fourth of the chicken on each of four plates. Top each with mango corn salsa and serve.

CHICKEN BURRITO WITH SALSA

Salsa has usurped ketchup as the most popular condiment in the United States, and it's easy to see why. Salsa is refreshing, spicy, fat-free, and incredibly healthy. In addition to fresh tomatoes, onions, and cilantro, salsa usually includes chile peppers. Chile peppers contain capsaicin, which can improve digestion, lower triglycerides, and reduce high blood pressure.

MAKES 4 SERVINGS

Cooking spray
½ cup fat-free refried beans
Four 10-inch flour tortillas
8 ounces cooked chicken breast meat
½ cup diced canned tomatoes with green peppers and onions, drained
½ cup shredded low-fat Mexican cheese blend
1 cup prepared salsa
2 cups shredded lettuce
1 cup chopped tomatoes
4 tablespoons nonfat sour cream

1. Spray a 9-inch square microwave-safe baking dish with cooking spray.

2. Spread 2 tablespoons refried beans on each tortilla.

3. Stir together the chicken and drained tomatoes in a small bowl and divide evenly among the four tortillas.

4. Top with 1 tablespoon cheese. Roll up and place in the baking dish.

5. Top with salsa and remaining cheese and microwave on high until hot and bubbly, 1 to 2 minutes.

6. Serve each person one burrito garnished with ½ cup lettuce, ¼ cup tomatoes, and 1 tablespoon sour cream.

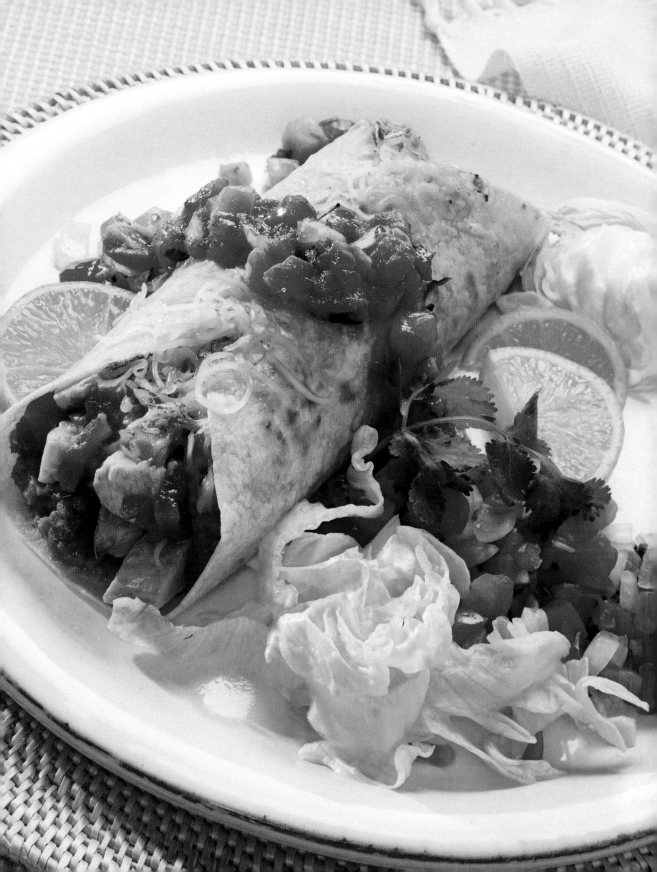

CHILI AND POTATOES

I prepared this dish for my good friend and client Al Roker on the *Today Show* as an alternative to his higher-calorie chili. The tomatoes, onions, and spices added to the prepared chili freshen the flavor, so you'll never know this chili came from a can.

MAKES 4 SERVINGS

4 red potatoes
Cooking spray
2 large onions, diced
6 cloves garlic, minced
One 32-ounce can crushed tomatoes
1 tablespoon ground chile, such as ancho or New Mexico
Three 15-ounce cans Shelton's® Turkey Chili
1 tablespoon paprika
½ cup plain low-fat yogurt
3 cups shredded cabbage
¼ cup low-fat Caesar salad dressing

1. Pierce the potatoes with a fork and place in a microwave-safe dish. Microwave on high until soft, 8 minutes.

2. Heat a medium saucepan over medium heat and spray with cooking spray.

3. Add the onions and garlic, and cook until translucent. Add the tomatoes, ground chile, the cans of chili, and paprika. Bring the mixture to a boil and reduce heat to low. Simmer the chili until flavors marry, 8 minutes.

4. Slice the potatoes in half and place two halves on each of four plates. Pour the chili over the potatoes and top each with 2 tablespoons yogurt.

5. Place the cabbage in a mixing bowl and toss with the Caesar salad dressing. Divide evenly among four plates.

6. Serve each person one plate of chili with one salad.

POTSTICKERS, BEANS, AND GREENS

Potstickers are Chinese dumplings that are panfried and then steamed, so one side is browned and crisp and the other is soft and tender. They're sold frozen and are delicious served with a soy or teriyaki dipping sauce.

MAKES 4 SERVINGS

2 teaspoons peanut oil
20 frozen chicken potstickers
¼ cup low-sodium chicken broth
4 cups frozen edamame (green soybeans in the pod)
Coarse salt
3 cups baby bok choy, leaves separated
1 tablespoon toasted sesame oil
1 tablespoon low-sodium soy sauce
1 cup prepared Asian dipping sauce

1. Heat a large nonstick skillet over high heat and add the oil. Bring a large pot of salted water to a boil.

2. Put the potstickers in the skillet and panfry, without moving, until the bottoms are golden and crisp, 4 minutes.

3. Pour the chicken broth in the pan and quickly cover to capture the steam. Reduce heat to low and steam until the dumplings are cooked through, 5 minutes.

4. When the large pot of water is boiling, add the edamame and boil for 3 minutes. Drain with a slotted spoon and season with coarse salt. Set aside and keep warm.

5. Pour out all but 2 inches of the water the edamame was cooked in. Put a steamer basket in the pot and add the bok choy leaves. Cover and steam for 2 minutes.

6. Remove from the heat and place the bok choy in a serving bowl. Drizzle with the sesame oil and soy sauce.

7. Divide the potstickers, edamame, and bok choy evenly among four plates. Serve each person one plate with ¼ cup dipping sauce.

TURKEY CUTLETS WITH LIME SAUCE

You can substitute the broccoli in this dish with any green vegetable you like, such as kale, green beans, or spinach.

MAKES 4 SERVINGS

1¼ cups low-sodium chicken broth
3 tablespoons dried minced onion
1 tablespoon dried parsley
One 5.7-ounce package plain couscous
2 cups broccoli florets
Cooking spray
Four 4-ounce turkey cutlets
½ teaspoon salt
½ teaspoon freshly ground black pepper
2 tablespoons minced garlic
¾ cup white wine
1 tablespoon lime juice, about 1 lime
1 tablespoon unsalted butter

1. Combine the chicken broth, 1 tablespoon of the onion, and the parsley in a medium saucepan over medium heat and bring to a boil. Stir in the couscous, cover, and remove from the heat. Let the couscous sit for 5 minutes and then fluff with a fork. Set aside and keep warm.

2. Combine the broccoli with 2 tablespoons water in a microwave-save dish. Microwave on high until tender, 4 minutes. Set aside.

3. Heat a large nonstick skillet over medium heat and spray with cooking spray. Season the turkey with salt and pepper and add to the skillet. Cook until no pink remains, 2 to 3 minutes on each side. Remove from the pan to a plate and tent with foil to keep warm.

4. Add the remaining onion, along with the garlic, wine, and lime juice to the pan. Bring to a boil and reduce heat to low. Simmer for 1 to 2 minutes. Swirl in the butter.

5. Put the turkey back in the pan and return the sauce to a boil to reheat turkey.

6. Divide the turkey among four plates and serve with ½ cup of couscous and one-fourth of the broccoli.

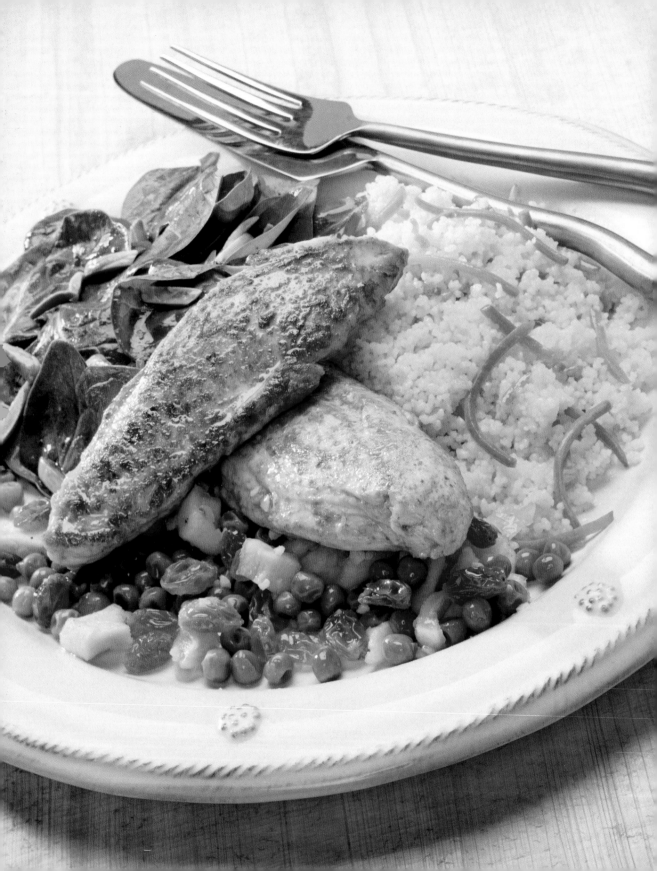

QUICK CHICKEN CURRY WITH COUSCOUS AND SPINACH SALAD

Couscous looks like small grains of rice, but it's actually tiny orbs of pasta. It's a staple food in Middle Eastern cooking and is often served with stews and curries. Try it in place of rice or potatoes for your next meal.

MAKES 4 SERVINGS

1¾ cups low-sodium chicken broth
½ cup shredded carrots
2 teaspoons minced garlic
One 5.7-ounce box plain couscous
Cooking spray
1 tablespoon curry powder
1 pound boneless, skinless chicken breast tenders
2 tablespoons dried minced onion
½ cup dried apples, chopped
1 tablespoon golden raisins
5 ounces frozen peas (half of a 10-ounce package)
6 ounces baby spinach
3 tablespoons slivered almonds
½ cup fat-free raspberry vinaigrette

1. Bring 1¼ cups of the chicken broth to a boil in a medium saucepan. Add the carrots, 1 teaspoon of the garlic, and the couscous. Cover and remove from the heat. Let sit for 5 minutes, remove the lid, and fluff the couscous with a fork. Set aside and keep warm.

2. Heat a large nonstick skillet over medium heat and spray with cooking spray.

3. Sprinkle the curry powder over the chicken, pressing it into the chicken with your hands. Add the chicken to the skillet and sauté until browned, 3 to 4 minutes.

4.   Add the remaining broth and garlic, along with the onion, apples, raisins, and peas to the chicken. Simmer over medium heat, stirring occasionally until heated through, 3 minutes.

5.   Meanwhile toss the spinach with the almonds and vinaigrette in a large bowl.

6.   Serve each person one-fourth of the chicken curry, ½ cup of couscous, and 1 cup of salad.

GRILLED ITALIAN CHICKEN

This chicken dish is reminiscent of chicken Parmesan but is much lighter. Instead of breading and frying the chicken before smothering it in loads of cheese, we've grilled it and topped it with a small amount of a very flavorful cheese blend. Grilled Italian Chicken is a perfect example of how to take a heavy, fattening classic and reduce the fat and calorie content to fit your diet. Try using the techniques in this recipe to lighten some of your other favorite dishes.

MAKES 4 SERVINGS

Cooking spray
1 pound thin chicken cutlets
2 teaspoons dried Italian seasoning
½ teaspoon salt
¼ teaspoon freshly ground black pepper
4 ½-inch slices Italian bread
1 teaspoon olive oil
1 teaspoon minced garlic
1 cup prepared marinara sauce
4 cups romaine lettuce

4 tablespoon fat-free Caesar salad dressing
½ cup shredded pizza cheese blend

1. Preheat the broiler. Heat a George Foreman–type grill and spray with cooking spray. Line a baking sheet with aluminum foil.

2. Sprinkle the chicken with the Italian seasoning, salt, and pepper. Place on the bottom half of the grill. Close and grill until cooked through, 3 to 4 minutes.

3. Meanwhile, place the bread on the baking sheet, brush with the oil, and spread with the garlic. Place under the broiler for 2 to 3 minutes until toasted. Remove to a plate and tent with foil to keep warm.

4. Pour the marinara sauce into a microwave-safe dish and microwave for 1 minute or until hot, stirring occasionally.

5. In a large bowl, combine the lettuce and salad dressing and toss to coat.

6. Remove the chicken from grill and transfer to the baking sheet. Top each piece with ¼ cup sauce and 2 tablespoons cheese. Broil until the cheese melts, about 1 minute.

7. Serve each person one-fourth of the chicken with 1 cup of salad and one slice of bread.

CHICKEN CORDON BLEU

Chicken Cordon Bleu is a rich French dish that rolls thinly cut chicken breast around ham and Swiss cheese before it is breaded and fried. Our light version omits the heavy breading and uses the broiler to melt the cheese instead of frying it in oil. The result provides you with all the delicious flavors of the original with a fraction of the fat and calories.

MAKES 4 SERVINGS

Four 2-ounce chicken cutlets
4 teaspoons olive oil
Two 1-ounce slices lean ham
Two 1-ounce slices Swiss cheese
4 cups mixed salad greens
2 cups diced pineapple (thawed if frozen, drained if canned)
¼ cup balsamic vinegar
4 small dinner rolls

1. Heat a grill pan or George Foreman–type grill to medium-high. Preheat the broiler. Line a baking sheet with aluminum foil.

2. Brush the chicken with the oil and grill until no pink remains, 2 to 3 minutes per side. Remove from the grill and place on the baking sheet.

3. Place half a slice of ham and half a slice of Swiss cheese on each piece of chicken.

4. Broil the chicken until the cheese melts, 1 to 2 minutes.

5. In a large bowl, toss the greens with the pineapple and vinegar. Divide evenly among four plates.

6. Serve each person one piece of chicken, one salad, and one dinner roll.

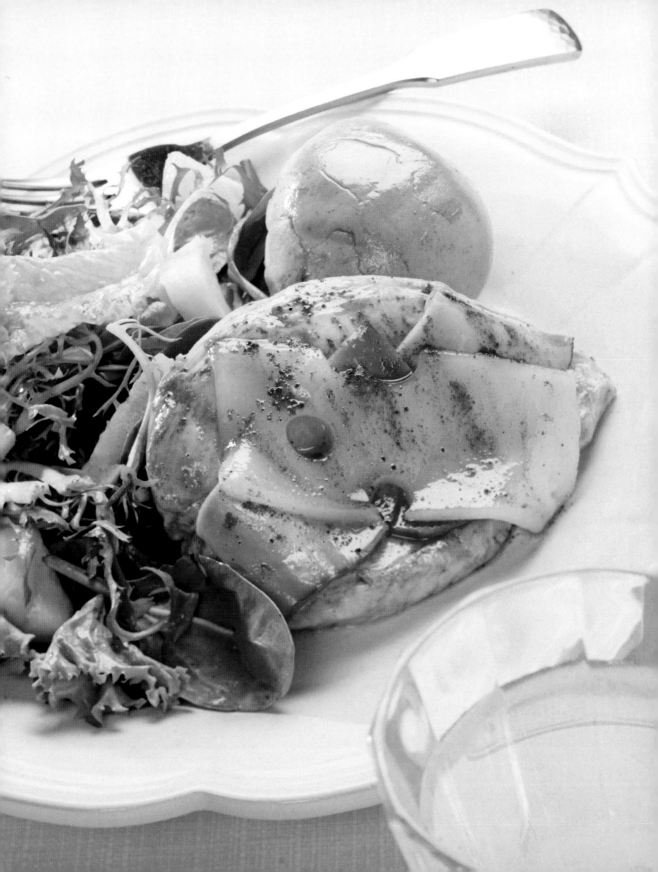

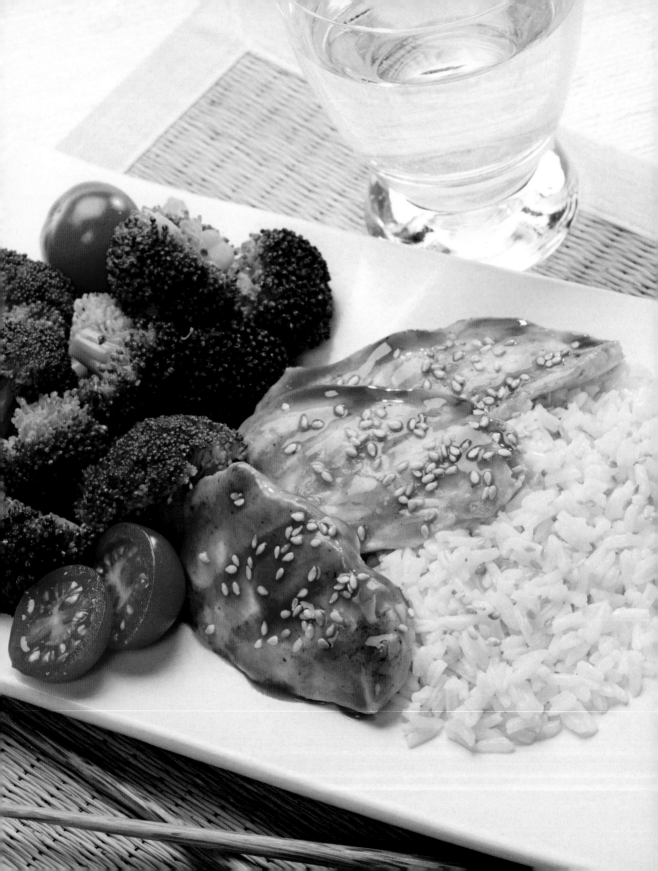

CHICKEN TERIYAKI

Your favorite bottled teriyaki sauce makes this dish a snap to get on the table quickly on a busy evening. Bright green broccoli florets and quick-cooking rice complete this delicious and satisfying meal.

MAKES 4 SERVINGS

Cooking spray
1 pound thin chicken cutlets
6 tablespoons prepared teriyaki sauce
2 tablespoons minced garlic
1 cup quick-cooking brown rice
10 ounces broccoli florets
2 teaspoons toasted sesame seeds

1. Preheat a grill or grill pan to medium-high and spray with cooking spray.

2. Combine the chicken with the teriyaki sauce and garlic in a small baking dish. Set aside to marinate while assembling the rest of the ingredients.

3. Combine the rice with 2 cups water in a medium saucepan over medium heat and cover. Bring to a boil and reduce heat to low. Simmer until the rice is tender and has absorbed all the water, 10 minutes.

4. In a large stockpot, bring 2 inches of water to a simmer and put in a steamer basket. Add the broccoli and cover. Steam until the broccoli is tender, 6 to 7 minutes.

5. Place the chicken on the grill and cook until the chicken is cooked through and the juices run clear, 2 to 3 minutes per side.

6. Serve each person one-fourth of the chicken and steamed broccoli and ¼ cup of rice. Garnish the chicken with sesame seeds.

CHICKEN SOUVLAKI

Souvlaki is a popular Greek food that consists of small pieces of lamb that have been marinated in olive oil, lemon, and oregano. For this recipe, we've used chicken instead of lamb to reduce the saturated fat while maintaining the intense flavors of the traditional marinade.

MAKES 4 SERVINGS

10 ounces cooked chicken breast meat
Zest and juice of 2 lemons
¼ cup low-sodium chicken broth
2 tablespoons extra virgin olive oil
1 teaspoon dried oregano
½ teaspoon minced garlic
Two 6-inch pita pocket breads
4 thin slices red onion
4 slices tomato
1 seedless cucumber, sliced
¼ cup nonfat plain yogurt
8 apricots

1. In a large zip-top bag, combine the chicken, lemon zest and juice, broth, oil, oregano, and garlic. Close the bag and shake gently to combine the flavors.

2. Heat a large nonstick skillet over medium-high heat.

3. Gently pour the chicken mixture into the skillet and bring to a boil. Reduce heat and simmer, uncovered, until heated through, 3 to 4 minutes.

4. Meanwhile, cut the pita pockets in half and heat in a microwave for 30 seconds.

5. Divide the chicken into four portions and stuff into each pita half. Top with the onion, tomato, and cucumber slices, and 1 tablespoon yogurt.

6. Serve each person one pita half with two apricots.

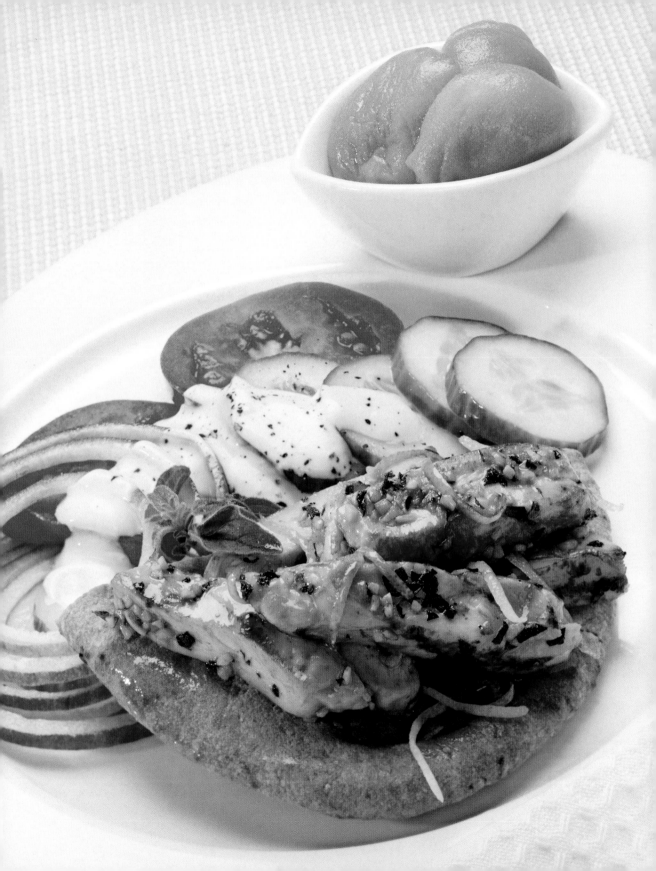

Chapter 9
MEATS

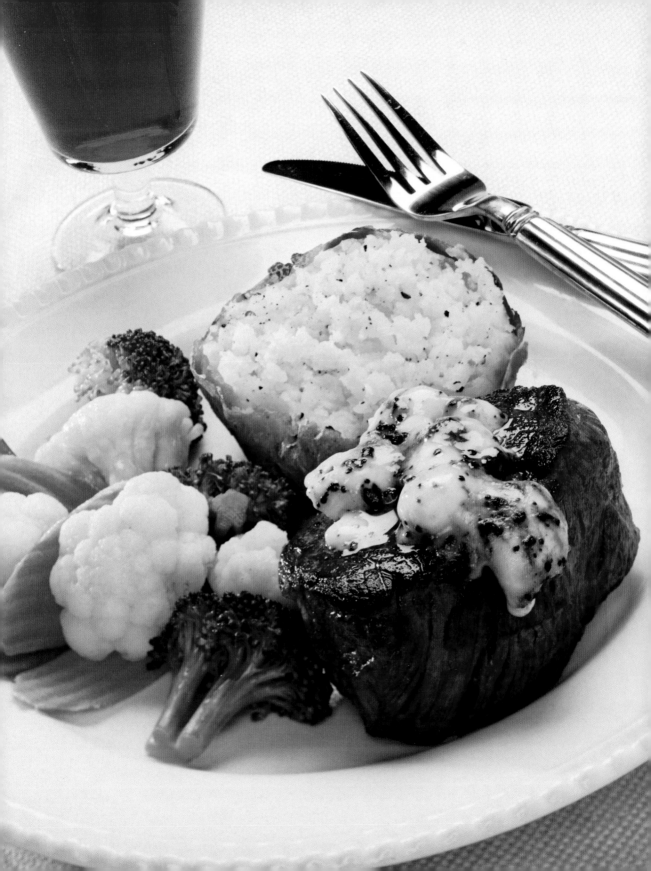

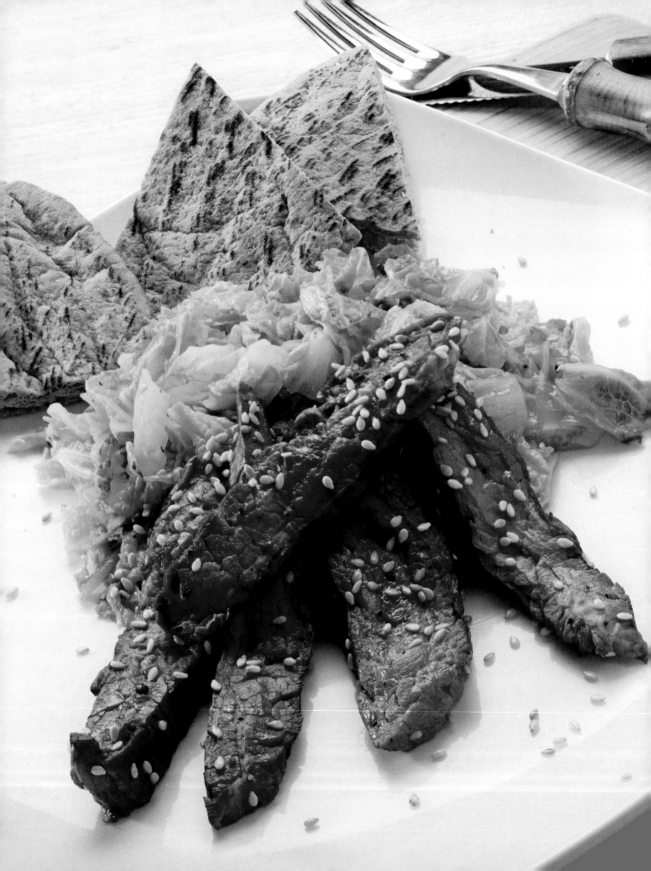

MARINATED FLANK STEAK

Flank steak is a long, thin, flat, and flavorful cut of beef. It's also known as London broil, which is technically a cooking method, not a cut of beef. Flank steak is well-suited to marinating, grilling, and broiling, but it can be tough. To ensure a tender piece of meat, cook it no further than medium rare, let it rest for five to ten minutes after cooking, and thinly slice it across the grain.

MAKES 4 SERVINGS

2 tablespoons Worcestershire sauce
1 tablespoon low-sodium soy sauce
Zest and juice from 2 limes
2 tablespoons minced garlic
¼ teaspoon cayenne pepper
1 pound flank steak
Cooking spray
4 cups Napa cabbage, shredded
1 tablespoon sesame oil
1 teaspoon toasted sesame seeds
2 pita breads

1. Stir together the Worcestershire sauce, soy sauce, lime zest and juice, garlic, and cayenne.

2. Place the flank steak in a large dish and coat with the marinade.

3. Preheat the grill or grill pan on high until it is very hot.

4. Grill the steak to desired doneness, 5 minutes per side for medium rare. Remove from heat, transfer to a large cutting board, tent with foil, and let rest for at least 5 minutes before slicing.

5. Heat a large nonstick sauté pan over medium-high heat and spray with cooking spray.

6. Add the shredded cabbage to hot pan and cook, stirring constantly, until cabbage just starts to wilt, 1 to 2 minutes. Remove from heat and stir in the sesame oil. Sprinkle with toasted sesame seeds.

7. Divide the cabbage evenly among four plates.

8. Cut the steak across the grain (perpendicular to the long fibers that run through the meat) into thin strips and arrange one-fourth of the meat on each cabbage salad.

9. Serve each person one salad with half a pita bread.

MEATLOAF PATTIES

Dividing meatloaf into individual patties significantly cuts down on baking time and offers more of what people love most about meatloaf—the crispy, browned crust!

MAKES 4 SERVINGS

4 teaspoons olive oil
1 pound lean ground beef
⅓ cup seasoned bread crumbs
1 egg, lightly beaten
1 teaspoon coarse salt
1 teaspoon freshly ground black pepper
2 teaspoons garlic powder
2 tablespoons low-sodium soy sauce
1 pound prepared baby carrots

1. Heat a large nonstick skillet over medium heat and add the oil.

2. In a large bowl, gently fold ground beef, bread crumbs, egg, salt, pepper, garlic powder, and soy sauce together and form into four patties.

3. Add patties to skillet and cook, turning once, until cooked through, 6 to 7 minutes per side.

4. Meanwhile, bring 2 inches of water to a simmer in a large stockpot and add a steamer basket. Add the carrots, cover, and steam 4 to 5 minutes or until tender.

5. Serve each person one patty and one-fourth of the carrots.

GRILLED BLACKENED SKIRT STEAK

Skirt steak is another long, flat piece of meat that is cut from the flank of the cow. It is usually marinated and grilled over high heat. To keep this cut tender, cook it rare, let it rest after cooking, and slice it across the grain.

MAKES 4 SERVINGS

2 teaspoons coarse salt
1 tablespoon cracked black peppercorns
1 teaspoon cayenne pepper
2 tablespoons minced garlic
2 tablespoons dried minced onion
1 tablespoon paprika
1 tablespoon olive oil
1 tablespoon soy sauce
1 pound skirt steak
4 small russet potatoes
4 cups mixed salad greens
½ cup cherry tomatoes, cut in half
4 tablespoons balsamic vinegar
4 tablespoons low-fat sour cream

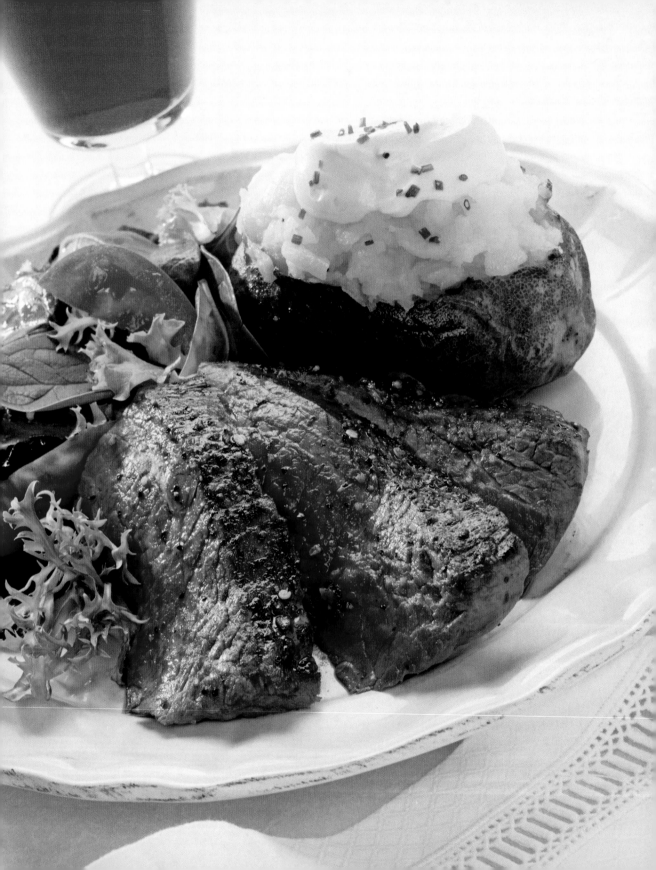

1. Mix together salt, peppercorn, cayenne, garlic, onion, paprika, olive oil, and soy sauce in a small bowl. Press spice mixture into both sides of the steak.

2. Heat a grill or grill pan on high until very hot.

3. Place the meat on the grill and cook to desired doneness, 3 to 4 minutes per side for medium rare. Remove from heat, transfer to a large cutting board, tent with foil, and let rest for 5 to 10 minutes before slicing.

4. While the steak cooks, pierce the potatoes with a fork and microwave on high until tender, 6 to 8 minutes.

5. In a large bowl, toss the salad greens with the tomatoes and vinegar. Divide evenly among four plates.

6. Thinly slice the steak across the grain and divide equally among four plates.

7. Along with the steak, serve each person one potato garnished with 1 tablespoon sour cream and one salad.

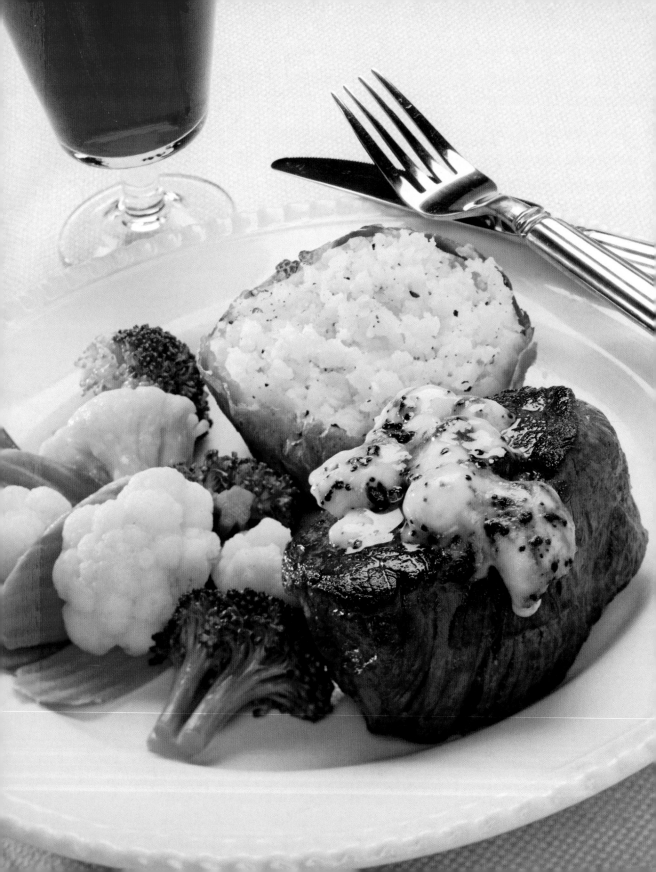

FILET MIGNON TOPPED WITH BLUE CHEESE, MIXED VEGGIES, AND BAKED POTATO

The tenderloin is the most tender cut of beef you can buy. Use quick cooking methods, such as broiling, grilling, or panfrying, to bring out this cut's ideal flavor and texture.

MAKES 4 SERVINGS

¾ pound beef tenderloin, cut into 4 pieces
⅛ teaspoon kosher salt
⅛ teaspoon freshly ground black pepper
2 cups mixed vegetables
2 medium russet potatoes
4 ounces crumbled blue cheese, about ½ cup

1. Preheat the broiler and season the filets with salt and black pepper.

2. In a large stockpot, bring 2 inches of water to a simmer and place a steamer basket in the pot. Add the vegetables, cover, and steam for 6 to 7 minutes.

3. Meanwhile, prick the potatoes with a fork and microwave on high for 3 minutes. Turn the potatoes and microwave for 3 minutes more, until tender.

4. Place the filets on a small baking sheet or broiler pan and put under the broiler. Broil to desired doneness, 3 minutes per side for medium rare.

5. Remove from the broiler, top the filets with blue cheese, and broil 30 seconds more to melt the cheese.

6. Serve each person one filet mignon, ½ cup of the mixed veggies, and half a baked potato.

BARBECUED FLANK STEAK WITH GRILLED VEGGIES AND RICE

Grilled vegetables are a delectable way to tempt carnivores to get some roughage in their diets. Seasoned with coarse salt, freshly cracked black pepper, and dried parsley, grilled squash takes on a sweet flavor and delicate texture that pairs beautifully with barbecued flank steak.

Makes 4 servings

1 pound flank steak
½ cup prepared barbecue sauce
1 cup quick-cooking brown rice
1 cup low-sodium beef broth
1 zucchini, sliced lengthwise into ½-inch slices
1 yellow squash, sliced lengthwise into ½-inch slices
1 red onion, sliced, rings kept intact
1 tablespoon olive oil
1 teaspoon dried parsley
½ teaspoon salt
¼ teaspoon freshly ground black pepper

1. Preheat the broiler. Line a baking sheet with aluminum foil.

2. Score both sides of the steak in a diamond pattern with a sharp knife. Place the steak on the baking sheet and coat each side with barbecue sauce.

3. Broil the steak to desired doneness, 6 minutes per side for medium rare. Remove from heat and transfer to a large cutting board, tent with foil, and let rest for at least 5 minutes.

4. Meanwhile, combine the rice and beef broth in a medium saucepan over medium heat and cover. Bring to a boil and reduce heat to low. Simmer until the rice is tender and has absorbed all the broth, 10 minutes.

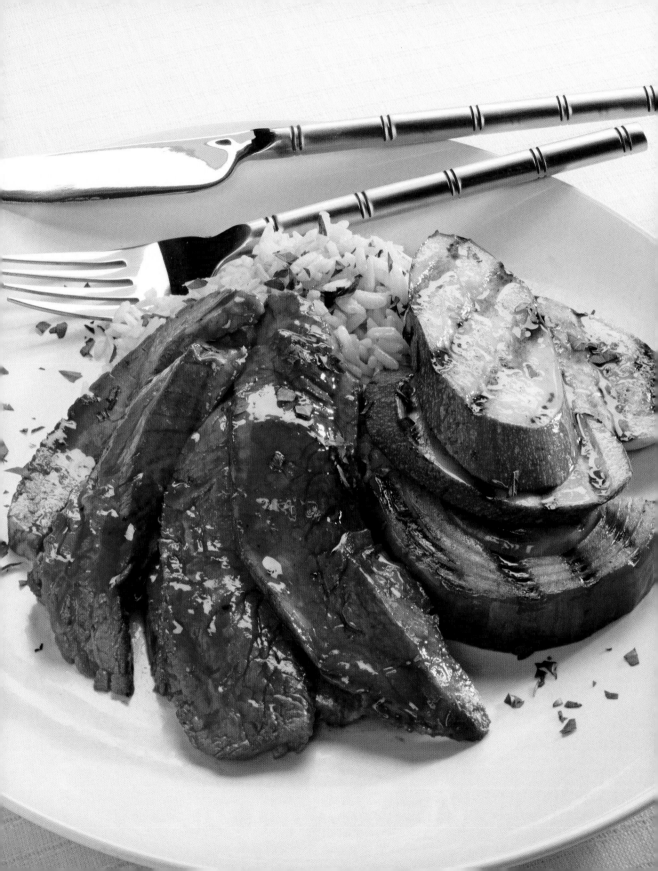

5. Carefully place the zucchini, squash, and onion on a baking sheet, brush with the oil, and sprinkle with parsley, salt, and pepper.

6. Place under the broiler and cook until the vegetables are tender and browned, 3 to 4 minutes per side.

7. Thinly slice the flank steak against the grain and divide equally among four plates. Serve each person ½ cup rice and one-fourth of the vegetables.

CHEESEBURGER PIE WITH MIXED GREENS

Regular ground beef usually contains 25 percent fat by weight; choosing extra-lean ground beef cuts the fat by 20 percent.

MAKES 4 SERVINGS

Two 6-inch pocketless pita breads
¾ pound extra-lean ground beef
½ onion, chopped
1 bell pepper (any color), chopped
½ teaspoon chili powder
¼ teaspoon salt
⅛ teaspoon pepper
4 ounces shredded cheddar cheese, about ½ cup
4 cups mixed salad greens
½ cup fat-free vinaigrette

1. Preheat the broiler. Line a baking sheet with aluminum foil.

2. Place the pitas on the baking sheet.

3. Heat a large nonstick skillet over medium heat.

4. Brown the ground beef in the skillet; drain off the fat.

5. Add the onions, peppers, chili powder, salt, and pepper to the ground beef and cook until the vegetables soften, 3 to 4 minutes.

6. Top the pitas with the ground beef mixture and sprinkle with the cheddar cheese.

7. Broil until the cheese melts, 2 to 3 minutes.

8. Meanwhile, toss the salad greens with the vinaigrette in a large bowl. Divide evenly among four salad plates.

9. Remove the cheeseburger pies from the oven, transfer to a cutting board, and carefully cut in half.

10. Serve each person half a cheeseburger pie with one salad.

GRILLED SIRLOIN STEAK WITH MUSTARD SAUCE, RICE, AND BROCCOLI

Sirloin steaks are typically lean, tender, and flavorful. Choose a steak cut near the short loin for the most tender steak.

MAKES 4 SERVINGS

1 cup quick-cooking brown rice
2 cups beef broth
2 tablespoons dried minced onion
Four 4-ounce sirloin steaks
1 tablespoon olive oil
½ teaspoon salt
¼ teaspoon freshly ground black pepper
4 cups broccoli florets
1 tablespoon slivered almonds
2 green onions, sliced
⅓ cup fat-free sour cream
⅓ cup fat-free mayonnaise
2 tablespoons spicy mustard
1 tablespoon prepared horseradish
1 packet artificial sweetener
1½ teaspoon vinegar
¼ teaspoon salt

1. Combine the rice, broth, and 1 tablespoon of the onion in a medium saucepan over medium heat and cover. Bring to a boil and reduce heat to low. Simmer until the rice is tender and has absorbed all the broth, 10 minutes.

2. Heat a grill or grill pan to high.

3. Brush both sides of the steaks with the oil and season with salt and pepper.

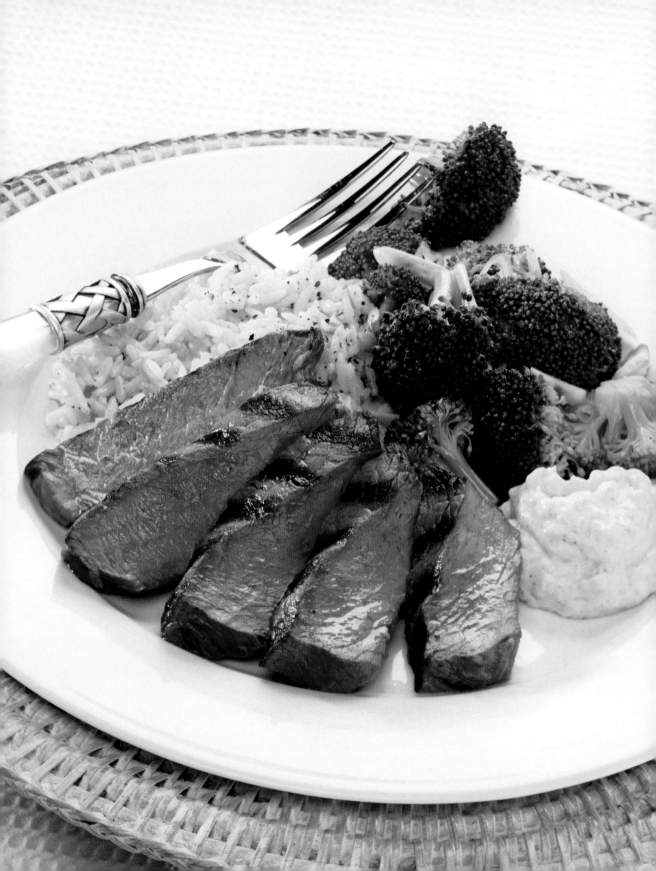

4. Grill the steak to desired doneness, 3 minutes per side for medium rare. Remove from the heat and tent with foil to keep warm.

5. Meanwhile, bring 2 inches of water to a simmer in a large stockpot and place a steamer basket in the pot. Add the broccoli, cover, and steam until tender, 6 minutes. Remove to a medium bowl and toss with almonds and green onions.

6. In a small bowl, whisk together sour cream, mayonnaise, mustard, horseradish, sweetener, vinegar, salt, and the remaining dried onion.

7. Serve each person one steak topped with one-fourth of the mustard sauce, ½ cup of rice, and 1 cup of the broccoli mixture.

GRILLED SIRLOIN PATTIES WITH ONION-MUSHROOM SAUCE AND COUSCOUS

This onion-mushroom sauce is smooth, rich, and utterly satisfying. Try this dish with rice or baked potatoes if you don't like couscous.

MAKES 4 SERVINGS

1¼ cups vegetable broth
One 5.7-ounce package plain couscous
1 tablespoon olive oil
1 onion, chopped
2 cups sliced mushrooms
1 envelope dried onion soup mix
1 tablespoon dried parsley
Four 4-ounce sirloin beef patties

1. Bring the vegetable broth to a boil and stir in the couscous. Cover and remove from heat. Let the couscous sit for 5 minutes and then fluff with a fork. Set aside and keep warm.

2. Heat a large skillet over medium heat and add the oil.

3. Put the onions in the skillet and sauté until translucent, 5 minutes. Add the mushrooms and cook for 2 to 3 minutes more. Stir in the soup mix and ½ cup water. Cook until the vegetables are tender and the sauce is thickened slightly, 3 minutes. Stir in the parsley.

4. While the vegetables cook, heat a grill pan or George Foreman–type grill. Grill the sirloin patties until no pink remains, 2 to 3 minutes per side.

5. Divide the couscous evenly among four plates. Top each with one sirloin patty and one-fourth of the onion-mushroom blend, and serve.

GRILLED PORK CUTLETS WITH CITRUS SALSA

We eat with our eyes before we ever take a bite of our food. That's why it's important that food look good as well as taste good. This dish is as visually appealing as it is delicious. The bright colors of the citrus salsa with lean pork cutlets brighten the plate as well as the palate.

MAKES 4 SERVINGS

2 cups packaged broccoli/cauliflower blend
4 thin-cut boneless pork loin cutlets, about 1 pound
¾ tablespoon olive oil
¼ teaspoon freshly ground black pepper
¾ teaspoon salt
One 15-ounce can mandarin oranges in juice, drained
One 15-ounce can crushed pineapple in juice, drained
¼ red onion, diced
2 tablespoons lime juice, about 2 limes
One 4½-ounce can chopped green chiles, drained
4 small dinner rolls

1. Preheat the grill pan or George Foreman–type grill to medium-high.

2. Bring 2 inches of water to a simmer in a large stockpot and add a steamer basket. Add the vegetables, cover, and steam until tender, 5 to 6 minutes.

3. Meanwhile, brush the pork with the oil and season with pepper and ½ teaspoon salt. Place on the grill and cook until barely pink in the middle, 2 to 3 minutes per side.

4. While the pork grills, stir together the oranges, pineapple, onion, lime juice, chiles, and the remaining salt in a small bowl.

5. Serve each person one pork cutlet topped with ¼ cup salsa, ½ cup of vegetables, and one dinner roll.

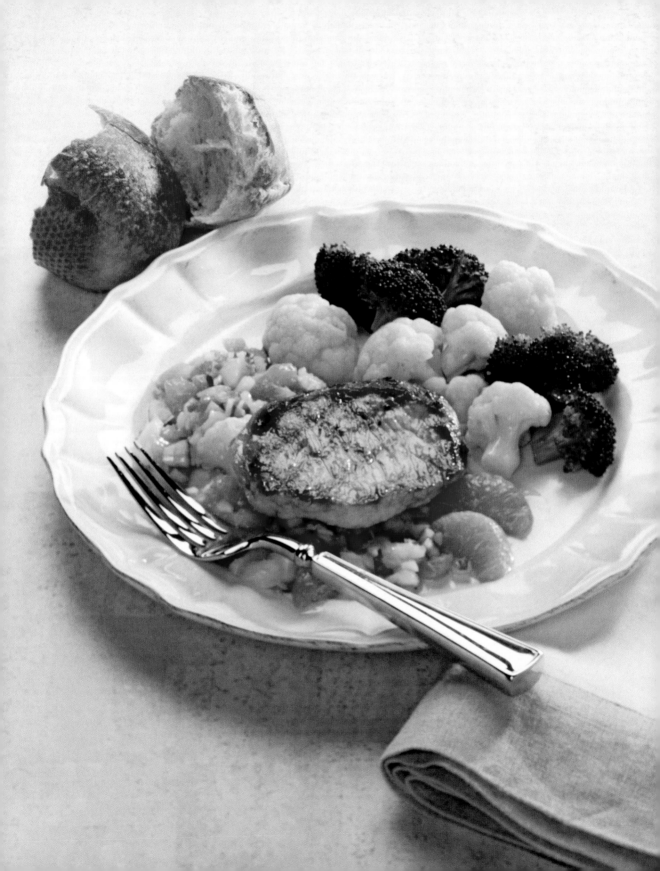

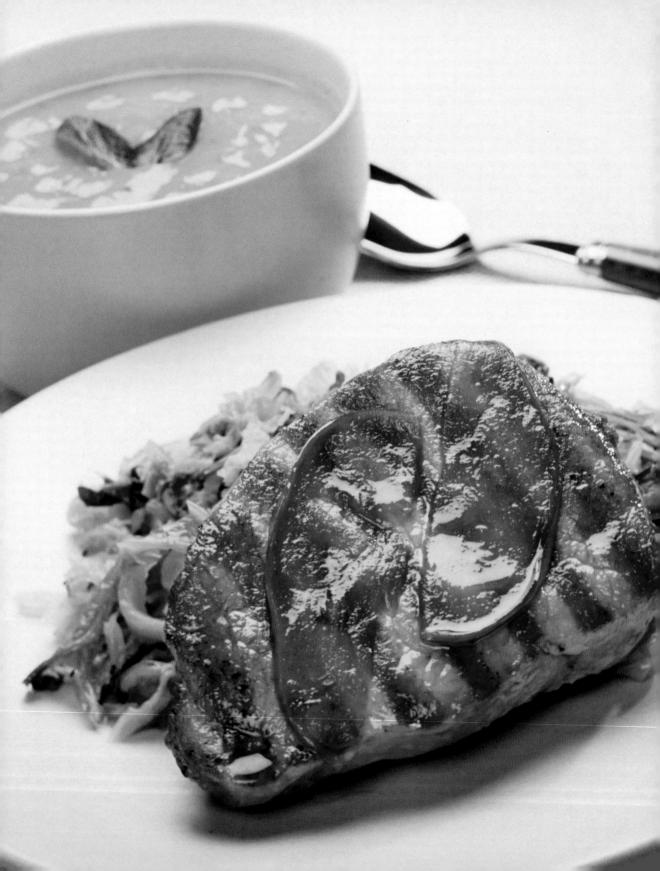

PORK CHOPS WITH SQUASH SOUP

Served with warm butternut squash soup, these tender baked pork chops are irresistible. We added steamed Napa cabbage for a light side dish. Feel free to substitute spinach if you prefer.

MAKES 4 SERVINGS

4 cups prepared butternut squash soup, such as Pacific Foods®
Cooking spray
4 thin-cut boneless pork loin chops, about 1 pound
Salt and freshly ground black pepper to taste
4 cups Napa cabbage, sliced into ribbons
1 to 2 tablespoons cider vinegar
¼ cup large sage leaves
4 medium apples

1. Put the soup in a large saucepan and bring to a simmer over medium heat.

2. Heat a grill or grill pan to medium-high and spray with cooking spray.

3. Season the pork chops with salt and pepper to taste. Place the pork chops on the grill and cook until barely pink in the middle, 4 to 5 minutes per side.

4. Bring 2 inches of water to a simmer in a large stockpot and place a steamer basket in the pot. Add the cabbage, cover, and steam until tender, 3 minutes. Remove the cabbage to a serving bowl and toss with the vinegar, adding salt to taste.

5. Spray a medium skillet with cooking spray and heat over medium-high heat. Add the sage and toast until crisp.

6. Serve each person 1 cup of soup garnished with toasted sage leaves, one pork chop, 1 cup of cabbage, and one apple.

PORK-AND-PINEAPPLE KEBABS WITH MIXED GREENS

Pork has a natural sweetness that pairs well with fruit, such as the pineapple in these kebabs. The corn and bell pepper salad is a perfect accompaniment to the kebabs—the bright yellow and red colors perfectly offset the color of the baby greens.

MAKES 4 SERVINGS

Cooking spray
4 metal or wooden skewers (soak wooden skewers in water for about 20 minutes
     before using to prevent them from burning on the grill)
1 pound pork tenderloin cut into 1-inch cubes
20 pineapple chunks (thawed if frozen, drained if canned)
½ cup Asian plum sauce
4 cups mixed salad greens
2 cups frozen corn kernels, (thawed)
½ red bell pepper, diced
¼ cup fat-free vinaigrette
1 tablespoon toasted sesame seeds

1. Heat a grill or grill pan to medium-high and spray with cooking spray.

2. Thread the cubed pork and pineapple alternately onto each skewer and brush
    with the plum sauce. Put the kebabs on the grill and cook until the pork is barely
    pink in the middle, turning to cook all sides evenly, 7 to 8 minutes.

3. Meanwhile, toss the salad greens with the corn kernels, the bell pepper, and
    vinaigrette in a large bowl. Divide evenly among four salad plates.

4. Remove the kebabs from the grill and sprinkle with sesame seeds.

5. Serve each person one kebab and one salad.

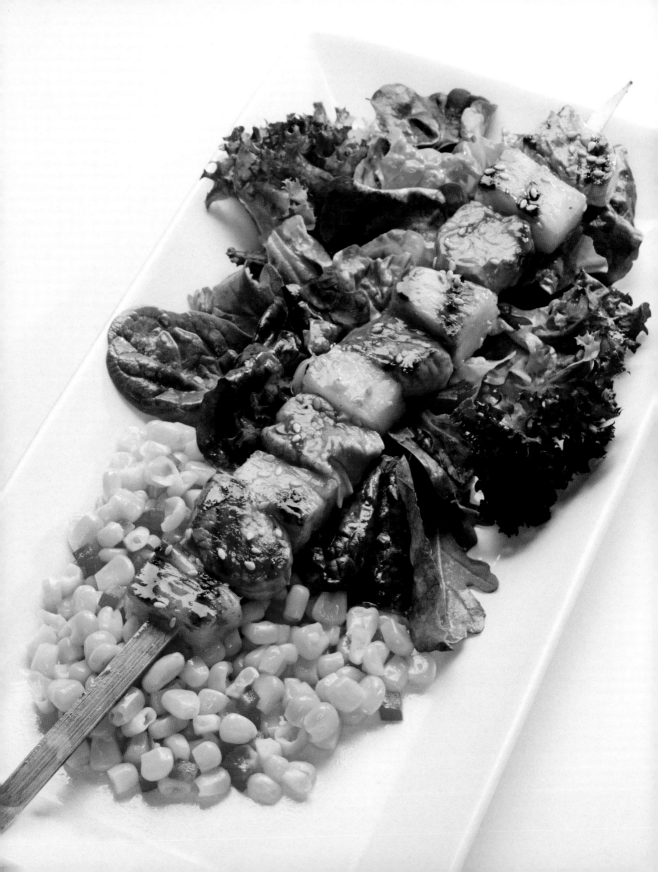

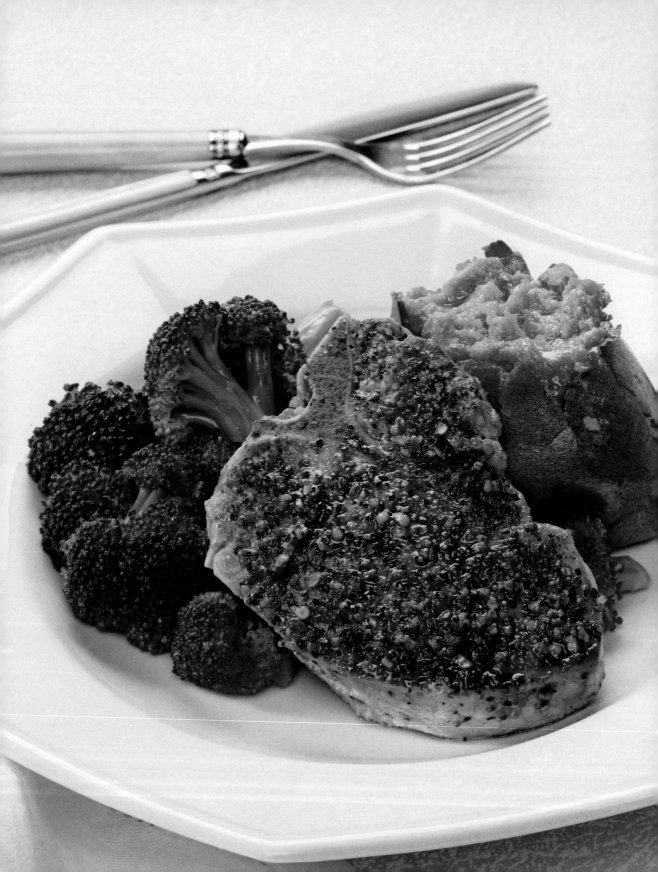

BLACKENED PORK CHOPS WITH YAMS AND STEAMED BROCCOLI

Yams contain vitamin B_6, which helps reduce the risk of heart disease. They also provide plenty of potassium, which keeps blood pressure down.

MAKES 4 SERVINGS

2 medium yams
2 tablespoons unsweetened apple juice
1 teaspoon cinnamon
Cooking spray
1 tablespoon olive oil
Four 4-ounce bone-in pork loin center cut chops
4 tablespoons Cajun seasoning, such as McCormick™
2 cups broccoli florets
½ teaspoon salt
¼ teaspoon freshly ground black pepper

1. Cut the yams in half lengthwise and place cut side down in microwave-safe dish. Pour the apple juice into the dish. Microwave on high until tender, about 8 minutes. Sprinkle with cinnamon, and set aside and keep warm.

2. Heat a large nonstick skillet over medium-high heat and spray with cooking spray.

3. Brush both sides of the pork chops with the oil and sprinkle with seasoning. Press the seasoning onto the pork with your hands. Place the chops in the skillet and cook to desired doneness, 3 to 4 minutes per side for medium.

4. Bring 2 inches of water to a boil in a large stockpot and place a steamer basket in the pot. Add the broccoli, cover, and steam until tender, 6 minutes. Season with salt and pepper.

5. Serve each person one pork chop with half a yam and ½ cup broccoli.

HONEY MUSTARD PORK CHOPS

Breaded pork chops satisfy meat lovers and carb lovers. Try this technique with chicken breasts if you prefer.

MAKES 4 SERVINGS

Cooking spray
6 tablespoons mustard
2 tablespoons honey
4 thin-cut boneless pork loin chops, about 1 pound
½ cup seasoned bread crumbs
4 teaspoons olive oil
4 cups broccoli florets

1. Preheat the broiler. Spray a baking sheet with cooking spray.

2. In a small bowl, stir together the mustard and honey and spread over the pork chops. Dredge the pork chops in the bread crumbs, coating both sides. Place the pork chops on the baking sheet and drizzle with the oil. Broil until brown on one side, 4 minutes. Turn the pork chops and brown the other side, 4 minutes more.

3. Meanwhile, bring 2 inches of water to a simmer in a large stockpot and place a steamer basket in the pot. Add the broccoli, cover, and steam until tender, 6 minutes.

4. Serve each person one pork chop and 1 cup of broccoli.

PORK TERIYAKI WITH COUSCOUS

Look for a low-fat soy- or ginger-based dressing for the salad that accompanies this pork teriyaki dish. The flavors in the teriyaki sauce will complement an Asian-style dressing.

MAKES 4 SERVINGS

1¼ cups vegetable broth
One 5.7-ounce package plain couscous
2 teaspoons minced garlic
¼ cup teriyaki sauce
1 teaspoon minced ginger
4 thin-cut boneless pork tenderloin cutlets, about 1 pound
4 cups mixed salad greens
½ cup low-fat salad dressing

1. Preheat the broiler.

2. In a medium saucepan, bring the broth to a boil. Add the couscous and 1 teaspoon of the garlic. Cover and remove from heat. Let stand for 5 minutes and fluff with a fork. Set aside and keep warm.

3. Mix the teriyaki sauce with the ginger and the remaining garlic. Brush both sides of the pork cutlets with the teriyaki mixture and broil until barely pink in the middle, 2 to 3 minutes per side.

4. Toss the salad greens with the dressing in a large bowl and divide evenly among four plates.

5. Serve each person one pork cutlet, ½ cup of couscous, and one salad.

GRILLED PORK WITH MANGO SALSA OVER RICE AND CARROTS

This mango salsa is a delicious combination of sweet fruit, pungent onions, and spicy jalapeños. Mix it up by substituting pineapple, papaya, or apricots for the mangoes.

MAKES 4 SERVINGS

1 cup quick-cooking brown rice
2 cups vegetable broth
4 thin-cut boneless pork tenderloin cutlets, about 1 pound
1 tablespoon olive oil
½ teaspoon salt
¼ teaspoon freshly ground black pepper
2 cups baby carrots
2 cups diced mango
½ small red onion, finely diced
2 tablespoons lime juice, about 2 limes
1 jalapeño chile, seeds removed and minced
1 tablespoon chopped fresh cilantro or 1 teaspoon dried cilantro

1. Combine the rice and vegetable broth in a medium saucepan over medium heat and cover. Bring to a boil and reduce heat to low. Simmer until rice is tender and has absorbed all the broth, 10 minutes.

2. Heat a grill pan or George Foreman–type grill to medium-high.

3. Brush the pork with olive oil and season with salt and pepper. Grill until barely pink in the middle, 2 to 3 minutes per side.

4. Meanwhile, bring 2 inches of water to a simmer in a large stockpot and place a steamer basket in the pot. Add the carrots, cover, and steam until tender, 5 to 6 minutes.

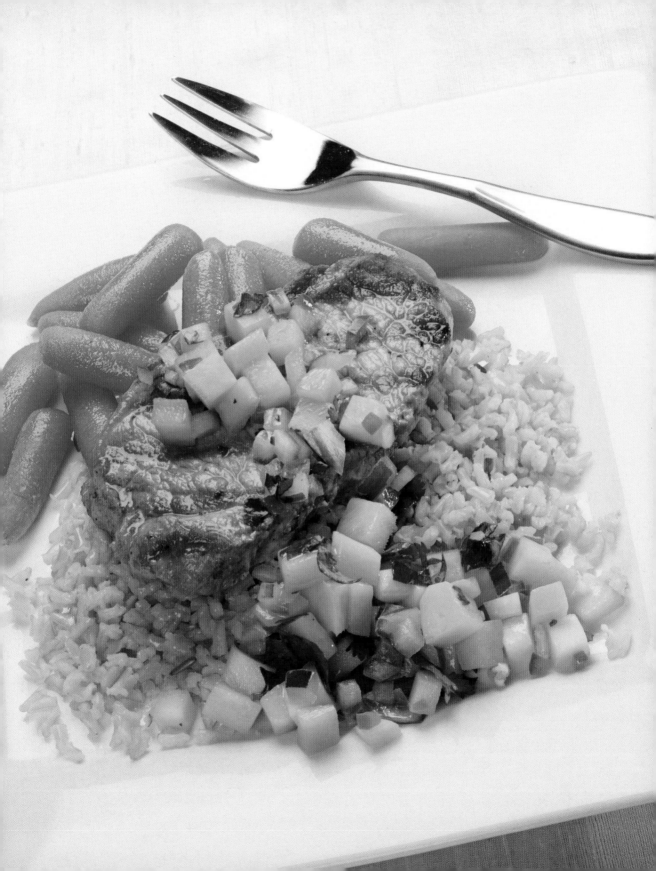

5. To make the salsa, toss the mango with the onion, lime juice, jalapeño, and cilantro in a small bowl.

6. Divide the rice evenly among four plates. Top with one pork cutlet and ¼ cup mango salsa. Serve with ½ cup carrots each.

APRICOT PORK OVER RICE WITH MIXED VEGGIES

Apricots are high in beta-carotene and lycopene, which makes them valuable in fighting heart disease. They also contain large amounts of vitamin A, which protects vision, as well as fiber to protect digestive health.

MAKES 4 SERVINGS

1 cup quick-cooking brown rice
2 cups low-sodium chicken broth
1 tablespoon olive oil
4 thin-cut boneless pork tenderloin cutlets, about 1 pound
Salt and freshly ground black pepper
½ onion, diced
½ cup dried apricots, diced
1 cup vegetable broth
2 tablespoons apricot preserves

1. Combine the rice and chicken broth in a medium saucepan over medium heat and cover. Bring to a boil and reduce heat to low. Simmer until the rice is tender and has absorbed all the broth, 10 minutes.

2. Meanwhile, heat a large nonstick skillet over medium-high heat and add the oil.

3. Season the pork with salt and pepper and add to the skillet. Cook the pork until browned and barely pink in the middle, 4 to 5 minutes per side. Transfer to a plate, tent with foil, and keep warm.

4. Reduce the heat under the skillet to medium and add the diced onion. Sauté until translucent and add the apricots and vegetable broth. Bring to a boil and reduce the liquid by half. Turn the heat down to low. Add the apricot preserves and stir to combine. Simmer until the sauce thickens, 2 minutes.

5. Add the pork back to the pan and coat with the apricot sauce. Heat the pork through, 2 minutes.

6. Divide the rice evenly among four plates and top each with one apricot pork cutlet.

Chapter 10
BURGERS, SANDWICHES & WRAPS

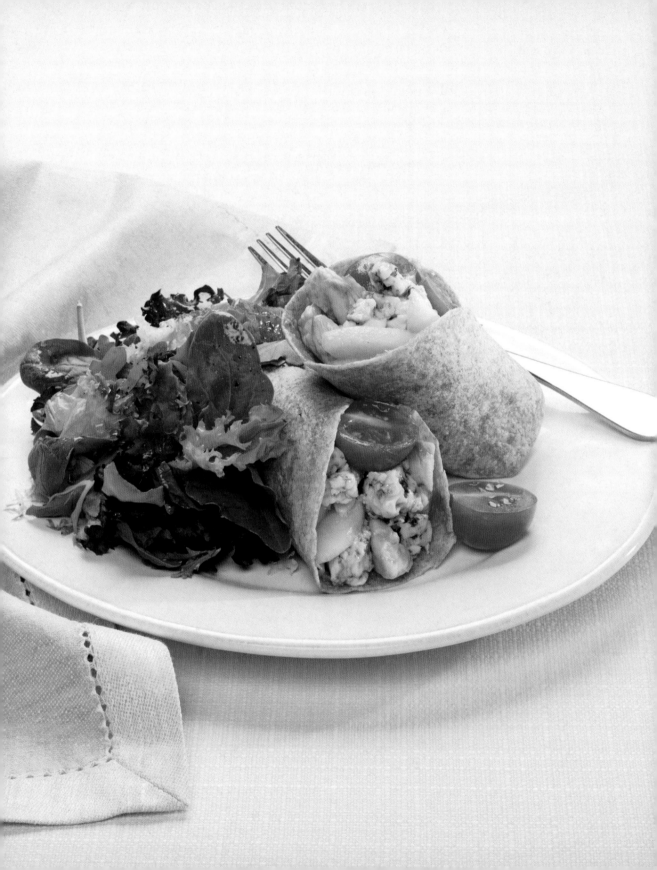

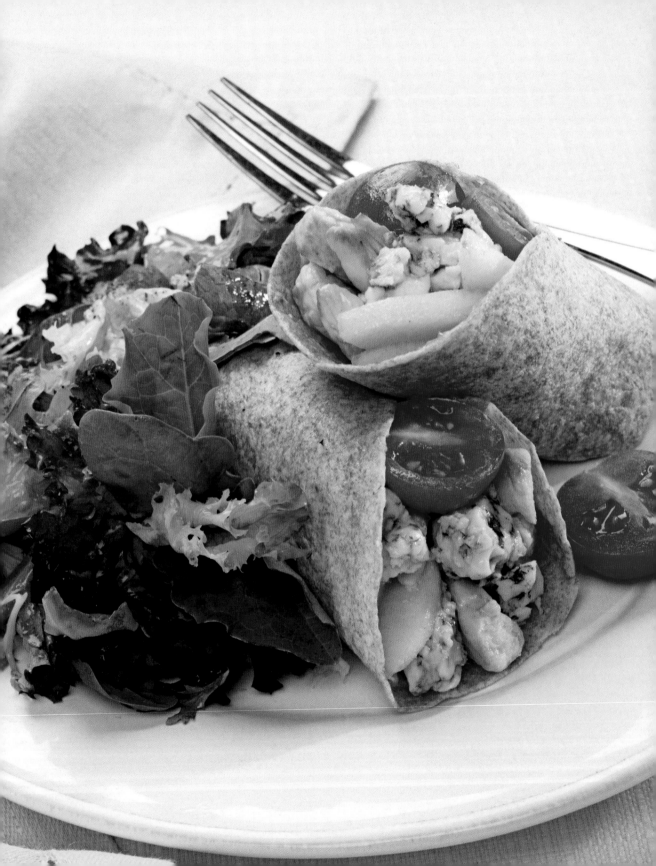

GRILLED CHICKEN GORGONZOLA WRAP

Gorgonzola cheese with pears is a classic flavor combination. Paired with a side salad, this chicken wrap makes a delicious and satisfying lunch or dinner.

MAKES 4 SERVINGS

8 ounces precooked chicken, diced
Four 6-inch flour tortillas
8 cherry tomatoes, halved
1 pear, cored and sliced lengthwise into 8 pieces
4 ounces gorgonzola cheese, about ½ cup
4 cups mixed salad greens
½ cup low-fat salad dressing

1. Evenly divide the chicken among the four tortillas. Top with the tomatoes, pear slices, and gorgonzola cheese. Roll into a burrito shape.

2. Toss the salad greens with the dressing in a large bowl and divide among four salad plates.

3. Serve each person one wrap with one salad.

ROAST BEEF AND SWISS CHEESE SANDWICH

This is a spin-off of the original Reuben sandwich, which includes corned beef and sauerkraut. Feel free to replace the beef with chicken or turkey—either would be delicious.

MAKES 4 SERVINGS

8 thin slices lean roast beef
4 slices Swiss cheese
½ cup onion sprouts
4 small whole grain rolls, sliced in half
4 tablespoons prepared Russian dressing
4 medium peaches

1. Place two slices of roast beef, one slice of cheese, and a small sprig of onion sprouts on the bottom half of each roll.

2. Spread the Russian dressing on the remaining halves of each roll and close the sandwiches.

3. Serve each person one sandwich with one peach.

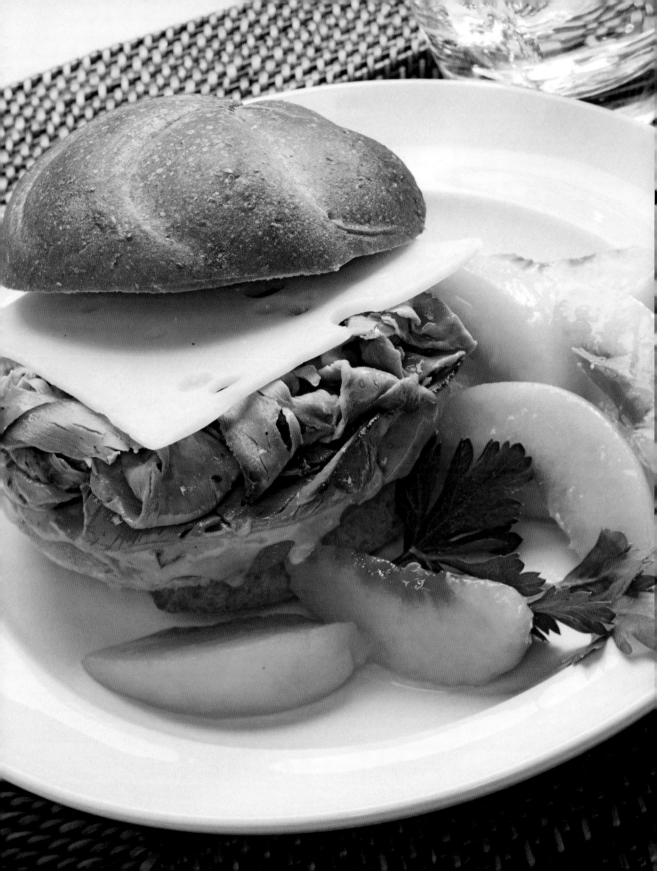

TURKEY SANDWICH WITH COLESLAW

A basic turkey sandwich is dressed up with an addition of prepared coleslaw in this unusual sandwich.

MAKES 4 SERVINGS

4 tablespoons mustard
8 slices whole grain bread
12 slices turkey breast
1 cup prepared coleslaw
2 cups raw baby carrots

1. Spread ½ tablespoon of mustard on each slice of bread.

2. Layer three slices of turkey on four slices of bread and top with ¼ cup coleslaw and the remaining slices of bread. Slice the sandwiches in half.

3. Serve each person two half sandwiches with a half cup baby carrots.

SMOKED TURKEY AND MOZZARELLA WRAP

Fresh mozzarella cheese is a delicious and unusual substitute for aged mozzarella. Its most common preparation is in a classic Italian salad, called caprese, a simple combination of summer-fresh tomatoes, basil, and fresh mozzarella. It's usually packaged in salted water and has a very light and refreshing flavor.

MAKES 4 SERVINGS

2 cups chopped romaine lettuce
½ cup low-fat Caesar salad dressing
8 thin slices smoked turkey breast
4 ounces fresh mozzarella cheese, diced
Four 10-inch flour tortillas
One 8-ounce jar roasted red peppers, drained and cut into strips

1. Combine the lettuce with the dressing in a medium bowl and toss to coat.

2. Layer two slices of turkey, 1 ounce of mozzarella cheese, and ½ cup salad on
    each tortilla. Divide the red peppers evenly among the tortillas. Roll the sand-
    wiches into a burrito shape and slice in half.

3. Serve each person two half sandwiches.

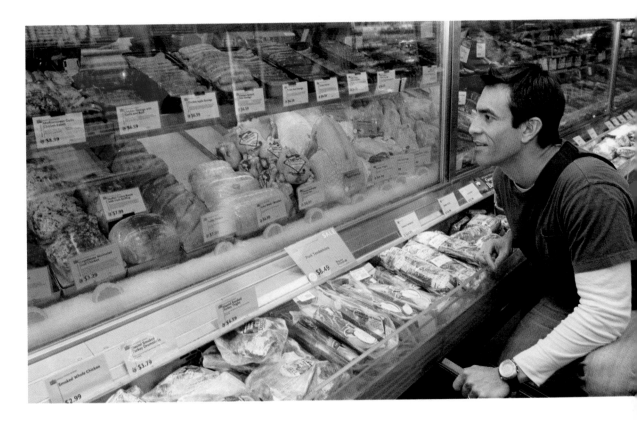

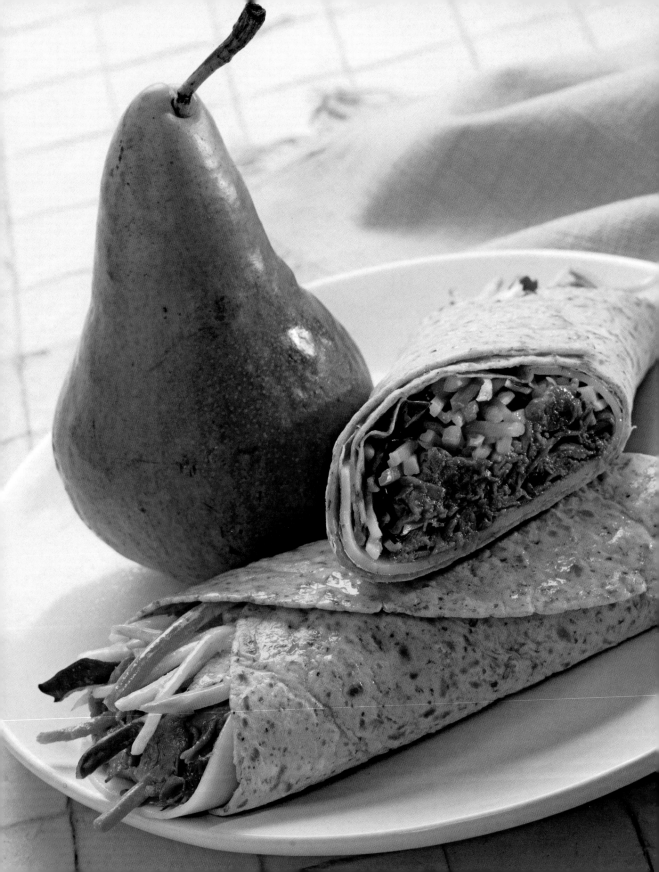

ROAST BEEF AND PROVOLONE WRAPS

Wraps are sometimes known as the "summer sandwich" and have recently gained popularity as the low-carb alternative to sandwiches made with bread. If you like horseradish, you'll love this roast beef and provolone wrap.

MAKES 4 SERVINGS

4 cups prepared broccoli slaw
½ cup low-fat horseradish salad dressing
Four 10-inch whole wheat tortillas
12 thin slices lean roast beef
Four 1-ounce slices provolone cheese
4 small pears

1. In a large bowl, toss the broccoli slaw with horseradish dressing.

2. Layer each tortilla with three slices of roast beef and one slice of provolone. Divide the broccoli slaw evenly among the tortillas. Roll into a burrito shape and slice in half.

3. Serve each person two half sandwiches with one pear.

PORTOBELLO MUSHROOM BACON CHEESEBURGER

Canadian bacon adds flavor and richness to this portobello mushroom "burger." Also called back bacon, it is significantly leaner than traditional bacon, because it is made from lean pork loin instead of fatty pork belly.

MAKES 4 SERVINGS

4 large portobello mushroom caps
4 teaspoons olive oil
¼ teaspoon freshly ground black pepper
¼ teaspoon kosher salt
2 sourdough English muffins, halved
5 cups mixed salad greens
4 slices tomato
Four 2-ounce slices Canadian bacon
Four 1-ounce slices Swiss cheese
½ cup fat-free balsamic vinaigrette
2 cups seedless grapes

1. Preheat the broiler. Line a baking sheet with aluminum foil.

2. Wipe the mushrooms with a damp paper towel to remove loose dirt. Brush with the oil and season with salt and pepper.

3. Place the mushrooms on the baking sheet and broil gill side up until browned and softened, 3 minutes, taking care not to burn. Turn over and broil an additional 2 minutes.

4. Meanwhile, toast the English muffins.

5. Top each muffin half with ¼ cup salad greens, one mushroom cap, one slice of tomato, one slice of Canadian bacon, and one slice of cheese.

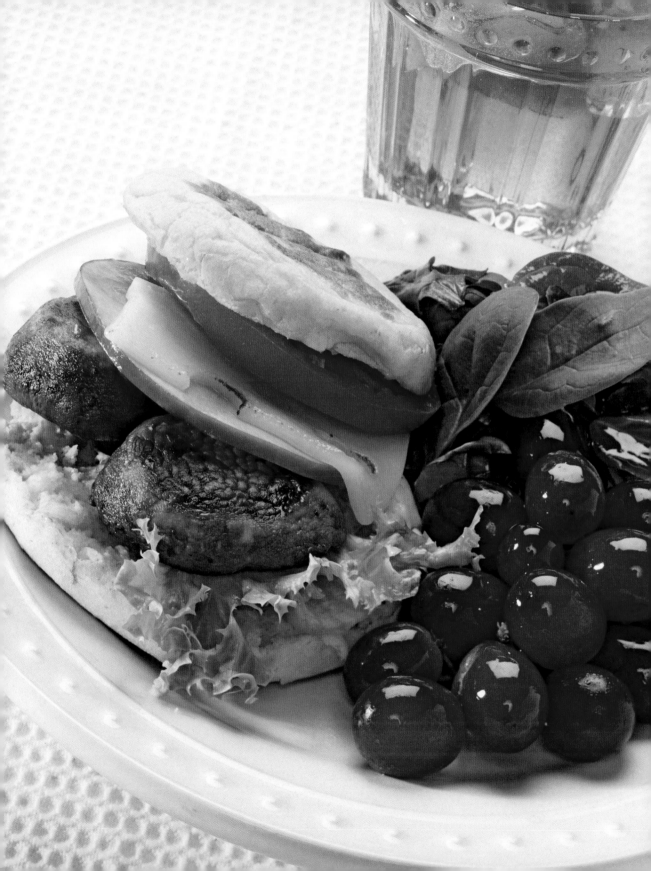

6. Toss the remaining salad greens with the dressing in a large bowl. Divide equally among four plates.

7. Serve each person one English muffin half with a salad and ½ cup grapes.

SLICED PIZZA BURGER

This meal satisfies every fast-food craving—it's a pizza and a burger! However, this drive-through trip won't derail your diet. Sirloin is a very lean, tasty cut of beef.

MAKES 4 SERVINGS

10 ounces ground sirloin
2 ounces part-skim mozzarella cheese, shredded, about ¼ cup
2 cups prepared pizza sauce
6 cups mixed salad greens
¼ cup low-fat salad dressing
4 small whole grain rolls, halved

1. Preheat the broiler.

2. Form the ground sirloin into four equal hamburger patties. Place patties on a self-draining broiling pan.

3. Broil the burgers until no pink remains, 4 to 5 minutes per side. Blot away any fat that accumulates on the burgers.

4. Top the burgers with cheese and pizza sauce and broil for 3 minutes more or until cheese is melted and sauce is hot.

5. Meanwhile, toss the salad greens with the dressing in a large bowl. Divide evenly among four salad plates.

6. Serve each person one burger on a roll with one salad.

MOZZARELLA CHEESE MELT

Pumpernickel is a type of sourdough bread made from rye flour. It's an excellent source of fiber and it helps fight colon cancer, gallstones, diabetes, and cardiovascular disease.

MAKES 4 SERVINGS

2 cups broccoli florets
4 slices lean ham
Eight 1-ounce slices part-skim mozzarella
4 slices tomato
8 slices pumpernickel bread
4 teaspoons unsalted butter

1. Bring 2 inches of water to a simmer in a large stockpot and place a steamer basket in the pot. Add the broccoli, cover, and steam until tender, 6 minutes.

2. Preheat a grill pan or George Foreman–type grill.

3. Place one slice of ham, two slices of cheese, and one slice of tomato between two slices of bread.

4. Spread ½ teaspoon butter on the outside of each slice of bread.

5. Grill the sandwiches until both sides are lightly browned and the cheese is melted, 3 minutes per side. Remove from the heat and slice in half.

6. Serve each person two half sandwiches with ½ cup of broccoli florets.

OPEN-FACED TUNA VEGGIE MELTS

These cheesy melts are a tasty alternative to plain old tuna sandwiches. Enjoy a cool spinach salad with mandarin oranges and almonds on the side.

MAKES 4 SERVINGS

One 6-ounce pouch or can tuna, drained
¼ cup low-fat mayonnaise
2 tablespoons pickle relish
¼ cup low-fat ricotta cheese
¼ cup shredded carrot
4 slices whole grain bread
4 slices tomato
Four 1-ounce slices cheddar cheese
4 cups baby spinach
One 15-ounce can mandarin oranges in juice, drained
1 tablespoon slivered almonds
½ cup fat-free vinaigrette

1. Preheat the broiler. Line a baking sheet with aluminum foil.

2. In a medium bowl, thoroughly mix the tuna with the mayonnaise, relish, ricotta, and carrot.

3. Spread the tuna mixture evenly on each piece of bread. Top with one slice of tomato and one slice of cheddar. Place on the baking sheet.

4. Broil the sandwiches until the cheese melts, 1 to 2 minutes.

5. Meanwhile, toss the spinach, oranges, and almonds with the vinaigrette in a large bowl. Divide evenly among four plates.

6. Serve each person one open-faced sandwich and one salad.

HOT CRABMEAT SANDWICH

Crabmeat is very perishable. Do not let it stand at room temperature any longer than necessary. Properly wrapped and frozen, it will keep for up to three months.

MAKES 4 SERVINGS

4 ounces fat-free vegetable cream cheese
2 tablespoons fat-free mayonnaise
2 tablespoons dried minced onion
½ tablespoon Worcestershire sauce
1 teaspoon hot sauce
6 ounces lump crabmeat
2 whole grain English muffins, halved
1 tablespoon slivered almonds
2 cups diced papaya (thawed if frozen, drained if canned)

1. Preheat the broiler.

2. Mix the cream cheese, mayonnaise, onion, Worcestershire sauce, and hot sauce in a medium bowl until well blended. Gently fold in the crabmeat. Mold the mixture atop the four muffin halves.

3. Broil the sandwiches until heated and bubbly, 3 to 4 minutes. Remove from the oven and sprinkle with the almonds.

4. Serve each person one English muffin half with ½ cup diced papaya.

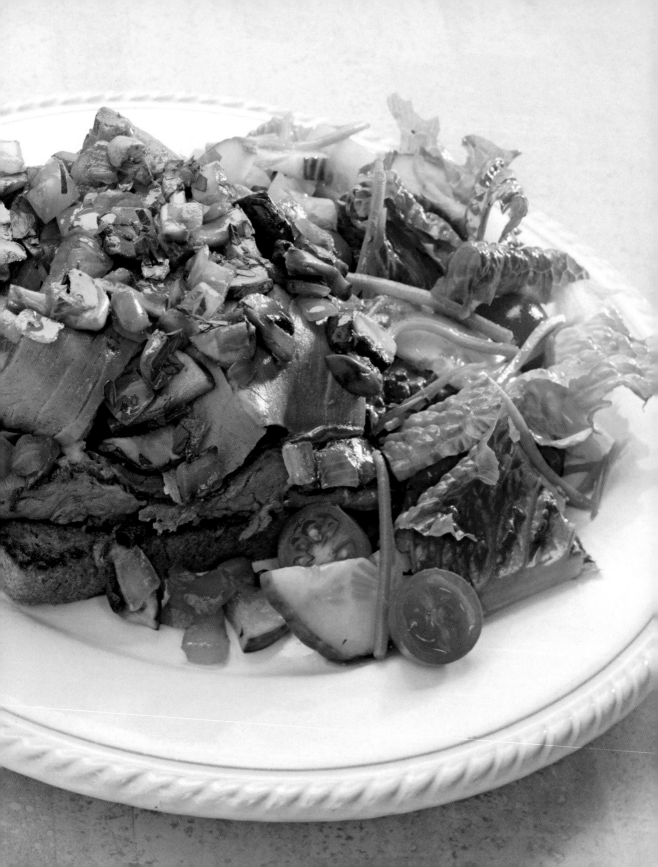

HOT OPEN-FACED ROAST BEEF SANDWICH

Thin, lean slices of beef are sautéed with onions and mushrooms to create a mouthwatering sandwich. A light vegetable salad rounds out this meal.

MAKES 4 SERVINGS

1 tablespoon olive oil
1 onion, chopped
½ cup sliced mushrooms
2 tablespoons onion soup mix
½ cup low-sodium beef broth
12 thin slices lean roast beef
4 cups romaine salad blend
1 pint grape tomatoes
1 cup shredded carrots
1 cucumber, chopped
¾ cup low-fat balsamic vinaigrette
4 slices whole grain bread

1. Heat a large nonstick skillet over medium heat and add the oil.

2. Add the onion and mushrooms to the skillet and sauté for 2 to 3 minutes. Stir in the onion soup mix and broth. Simmer for 2 minutes. Add the roast beef and simmer 1 to 2 minutes more or until heated through.

3. Meanwhile, toss the salad blend with the tomatoes, carrots, cucumber, and dressing in a large bowl. Divide evenly among four salad plates.

4. Toast the bread and place one slice on each of four plates.

5. Place three slices of roast beef on each piece of toast. Spoon the pan juices and mushrooms over the sandwiches.

6. Serve each person one sandwich and one salad.

TUNA SANDWICH AND TOMATO SOUP

We've combined two of everyone's all-time favorite dishes and created a simple, balanced meal. Take pleasure in tomato soup and a tuna sandwich and know you're eating right.

MAKES 4 SERVINGS

6 cups prepared roasted red pepper and tomato soup, such as Pacific Foods®
One 12-ounce pouch or can water-packed tuna, drained
3 tablespoons extra virgin olive oil
4 tablespoons lemon juice, about 2 lemons
Salt and freshly ground black pepper to taste
¼ cup finely chopped red onion
¼ cup finely chopped green onion
4 slices whole grain bread
1 cup baby spinach
4 pickles

1. Heat the soup in a medium saucepan over medium heat and bring to a boil.

2. Meanwhile, mix the tuna, oil, lemon juice, salt, pepper, and onions in a medium bowl.

3. Spread the tuna salad evenly on two pieces of bread. Top with the spinach and remaining two slices of bread. Cut the sandwiches in half.

4. Divide the soup equally into four bowls.

5. Serve each person one half tuna sandwich, one bowl of soup, and one pickle.

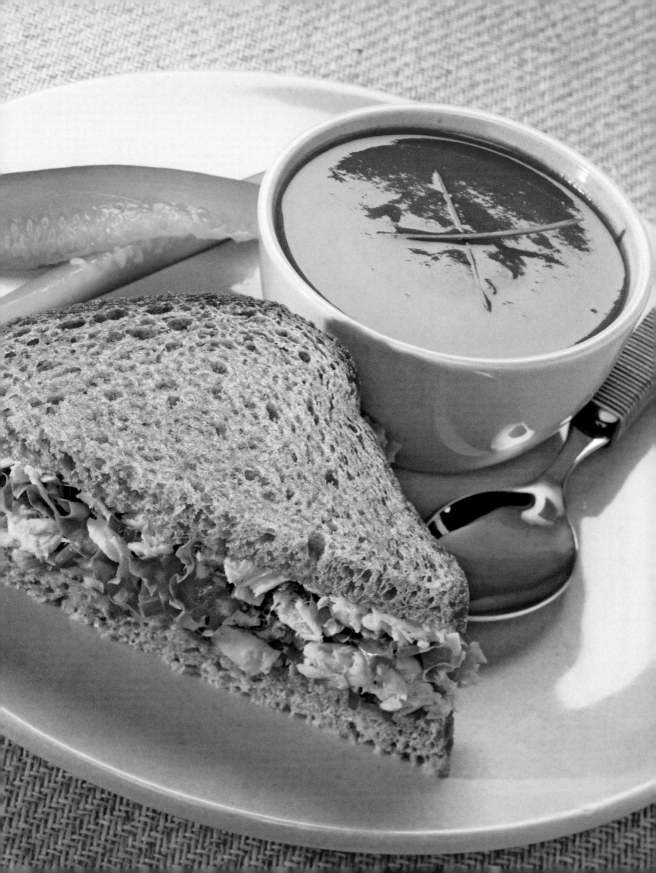

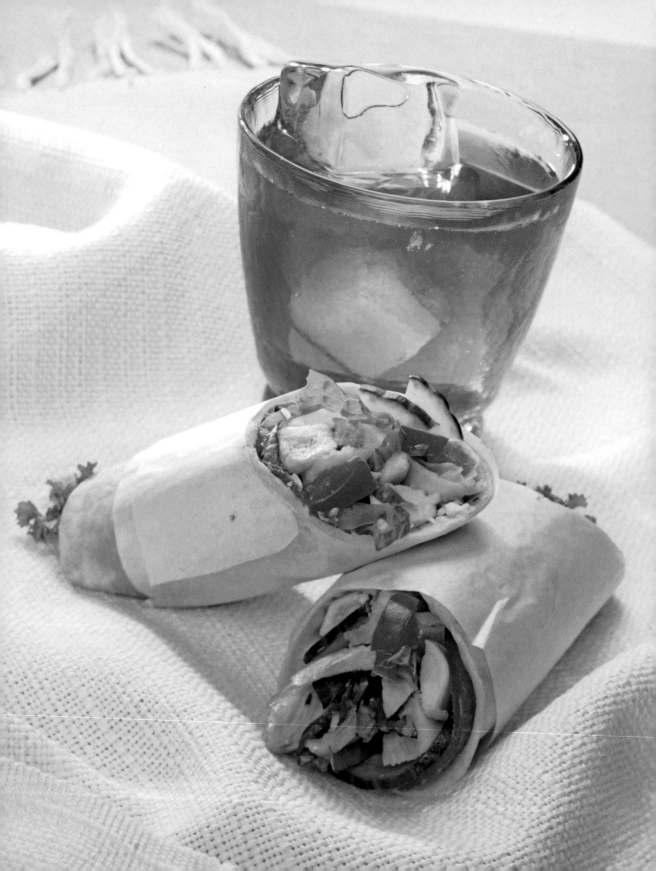

GREEK CHICKEN WRAP

Feta cheese is deliciously salty and pungent, which means that you don't have to use a lot of it to enjoy its flavor. If feta is too strongly flavored for you, try substituting with ricotta salata—an aged ricotta cheese that has a similar texture to feta.

MAKES 4 SERVINGS

Four 6-inch flour tortillas
½ cup low-fat ranch dressing
8 ounces cooked chicken breast meat, diced
1 cup shredded romaine lettuce
½ cup chopped tomato
½ cup sliced cucumber
4 ounces crumbled feta cheese, about ½ cup

1. Spread each tortilla with 2 tablespoons ranch dressing.

2. Divide the chicken, romaine, tomato, cucumber, and feta equally among the tortillas.

3. Roll into a burrito shape. Serve each person one sandwich.

MAHIMAHI WITH SWEET ONION SANDWICH

Mahimahi, also known as dorado, is a species of surface-dwelling fish found in tropical and subtropical waters. It's become quite popular and is sometimes eaten as a substitute for swordfish because of its firm texture and sweet flavor.

MAKES 4 SERVINGS

Four 4-ounce mahimahi fillets
4 teaspoons olive oil
½ teaspoon salt
1 teaspoon freshly ground black pepper
2 teaspoons garlic powder
2 tablespoons lemon juice, about 1 lemon
¼ cup fat-free mayonnaise
1 tablespoon pickle relish
1 teaspoon prepared horseradish
4 onion rolls, halved
Four ½-inch-thick slices Vidalia onion (or another sweet onion like Maui or Walla Walla)
4 slices tomato
½ cup mixed salad greens

1. Heat a George Foreman–type grill to medium-high.

2. Brush the fish fillets with the oil and sprinkle with salt, pepper, and garlic powder. Place on bottom of grill, close top, and cook until fish flakes easily with a fork, 6 to 7 minutes. Pour lemon juice over the fish.

3. In a small bowl, stir together the mayonnaise, relish, and horseradish and spread equally on the onion rolls.

4. Place the onion, tomato, and salad greens on the bottom of the rolls. Top with the fish and bun top and serve.

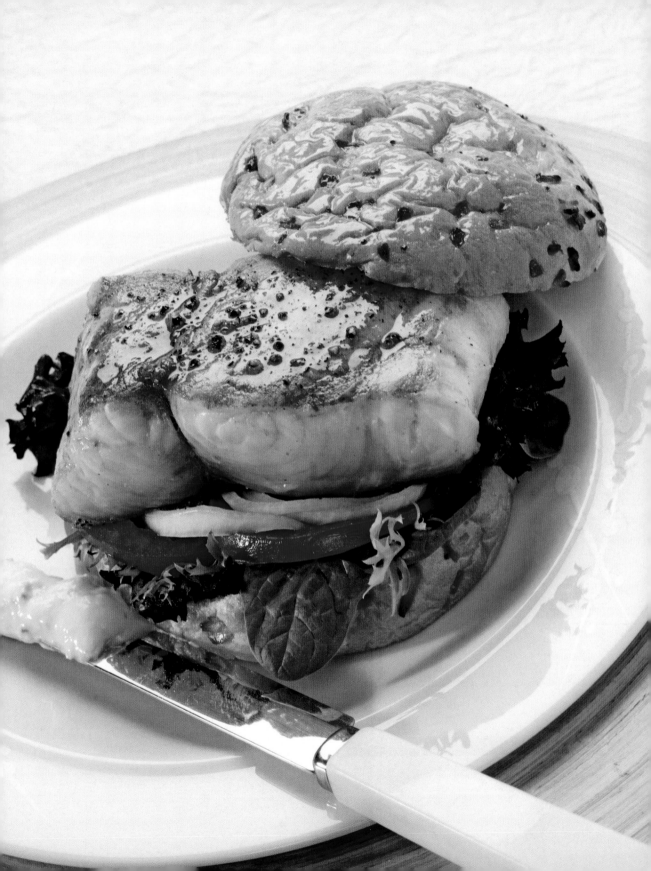

BARBECUED TURKEY BURGER

This juicy, flavor-filled barbecued turkey burger is perfect for everyday dinners or special occasions, such as the Fourth of July. To vary this dish, try using ground chicken instead of turkey.

Makes 4 servings

2 tablespoons low-sodium soy sauce
¼ cup prepared barbecue sauce
Four 4-ounce frozen uncooked white meat turkey burgers
4 onion rolls, halved
1 tomato, sliced
½ red onion, sliced
4 cups mixed salad greens
¼ cup low-fat salad dressing

1. Heat a grill pan or George Foreman–type grill to medium and spray with cooking spray.

2. Stir together the soy sauce and barbecue sauce in a small bowl.

3. Grill the turkey burgers until cooked through, 5 to 6 minutes per side. Remove from heat and brush with the barbecue-soy mixture.

4. Place each turkey burger on the bottom half of an onion roll and top with the tomato, onion, and bun top.

5. Toss the salad greens with the dressing in a large bowl. Divide evenly among four salad plates.

6. Serve each person one turkey burger with one salad.

TURKEY TORTILLA WRAP

Turkey is an excellent source of selenium, a trace mineral that's important to thyroid hormone metabolism, antioxidant processes, and immune system function. Studies have also found that people who eat diets high in selenium have lower incidences of cancer.

MAKES 4 SERVINGS

Four 6-inch whole wheat tortillas
12 ounces thinly sliced turkey breast
1 cup baby spinach
¾ cup prepared salsa
½ avocado, sliced into 8 slices
3 cups prepared broccoli slaw
3 tablespoons vinaigrette salad dressing
4 kiwifruit

1. Wrap tortillas in damp paper towels and soften in the microwave, 30 seconds.

2. Add 3 ounces of turkey, ¼ cup of spinach, 3 tablespoons of salsa, and two slices of avocado to each tortilla and roll into a burrito shape.

3. Toss the broccoli slaw with the dressing in a separate bowl.

4. Serve each person one wrap with one-fourth of the broccoli slaw and one kiwifruit.

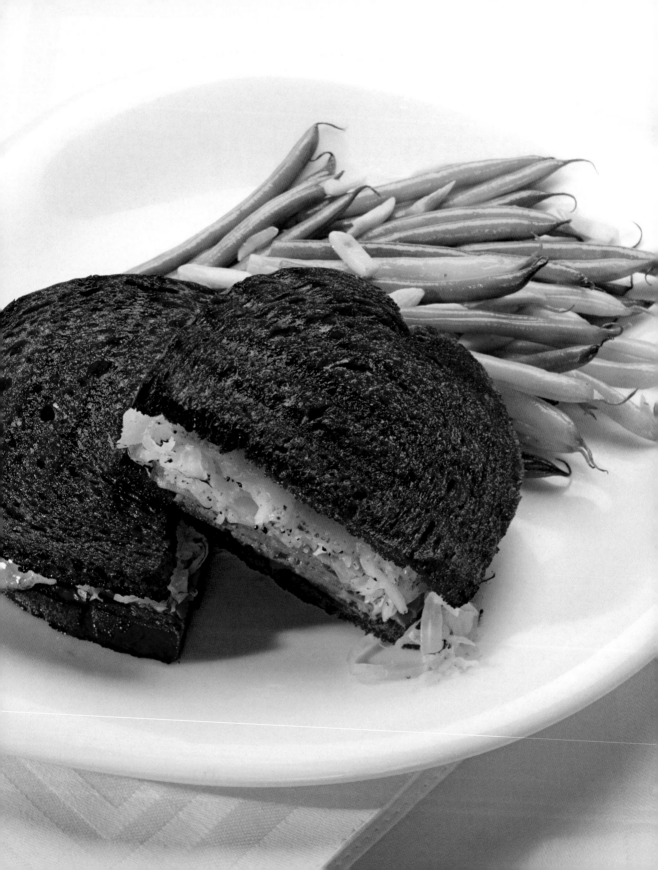

GRILLED REUBEN WITH BEAN SALAD

Corned beef is a formerly tough cut of meat, usually brisket or round, that's cured in a seasoned brine. When thinly sliced, it can be a deliciously flavorful and tender addition to a hot or cold sandwich.

MAKES 4 SERVINGS

Cooking spray
8 slices low-calorie rye bread
¼ cup fat-free Thousand Island dressing
8 thin slices lean corned beef
Four 1-ounce slices Swiss cheese
1 cup sauerkraut, drained
2 cups green beans
2 cups yellow wax beans
½ cup fat-free Italian dressing
2 tablespoons slivered almonds

1. Heat a George Foreman–type grill to medium and spray with cooking spray.

2. Spread each piece of bread with ½ tablespoon dressing. Divide the corned beef, cheese, and sauerkraut among four slices of bread and top with remaining slices.

3. Place sandwiches on the bottom of the grill, close, and cook for 3 to 4 minutes or until browned on both sides and the cheese is melted.

4. Bring 2 inches of water to a simmer in a large stockpot and add a steamer basket. Add the beans and steam until tender, 5 to 6 minutes. Remove the steamer basket from the pot and run under cold water to chill the beans. Dry on paper towels.

5. In a large bowl, toss the beans with the dressing. Top with almonds.

6. Cut the sandwiches in half and serve each person two half sandwiches with one-fourth of the bean salad.

SALMON BURGERS AND SUGAR SNAP PEAS

Salmon is low in calories and saturated fat but high in protein and healthy omega-3 fatty acids. Salmon also offers a lot of niacin, vitamin B_6, and vitamin B_{12}.

MAKES 4 SERVINGS

4 frozen salmon burgers
3 cups sugar snap peas
4 whole grain hamburger buns
4 tablespoons mustard
4 tablespoons fat-free mayonnaise
1 cup baby spinach
3 cups grapes

1. Heat a grill pan or George Foreman–type grill to medium.

2. Place the frozen salmon burgers on the grill and close the lid. Grill until cooked through, 8 to 10 minutes.

3. Bring 2 inches of water to a simmer in a large stockpot and place a steamer basket in the pot. Add the sugar snaps, cover, and steam until tender, 2 minutes.

4. Slather the hamburger buns with 1 tablespoon each mustard and mayonnaise. Add the salmon burgers to the buns and top each with ¼ cup spinach.

5. Serve each person one salmon burger with ¾ cup grapes on the side.

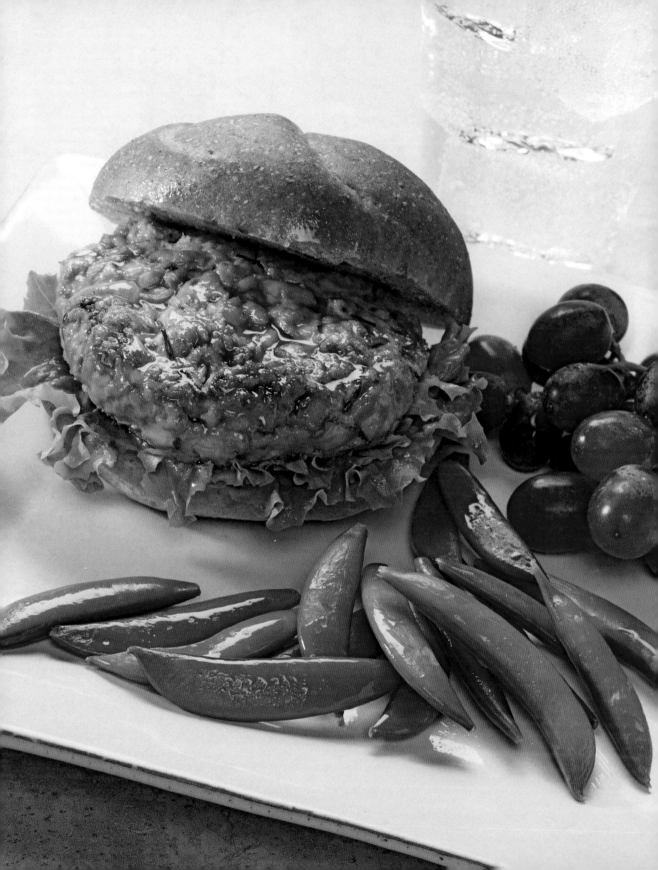

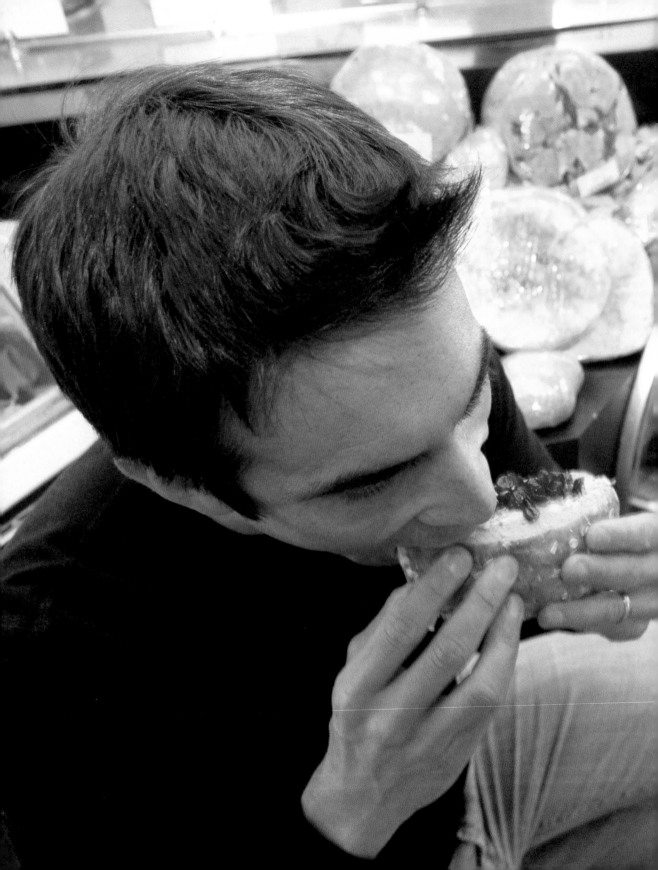

TURKEY AND CRANBERRY SANDWICH

This turkey, cream cheese, and cranberry sauce trio revives Thanksgiving cravings anytime of year. Use leftover turkey from Thanksgiving or turkey from the deli to make these sandwiches quickly and easily.

MAKES 4 SERVINGS

½ cup low-fat cream cheese
8 slices whole grain bread
½ cup cranberry sauce
8 ounces sliced turkey breast
4 large lettuce leaves
3 cups baby carrots

1. Spread 2 tablespoons cream cheese on four slices of bread and 2 tablespoons cranberry sauce on the remaining slices of bread. Add the turkey and lettuce and close the sandwich. Slice sandwiches in half.

2. Serve each person two half sandwiches with ¾ cup carrots.

HONEY MUSTARD HAM PITA

Sweet, tangy honey mustard dresses up this ham pita sandwich, making it a sensational lunch or dinnertime favorite.

MAKES 4 SERVINGS

6 tablespoons honey mustard dressing
4 whole grain pita pocket breads, halved
Eight 1-ounce slices lean ham
Four 1-ounce slices Swiss cheese
2 cups baby spinach
2 cups carrot sticks

1. Spread honey mustard dressing inside each pita pocket half.

2. Stuff each pocket with one slice of ham, one slice of cheese, and ½ cup of spinach.

3. Serve each person two sandwich halves with ½ cup carrot sticks on the side.

STUFFED BURGERS

Worcestershire sauce and blue cheese crumbles add a tangy kick to these burgers that taste best when grilled. Enjoy sweet summer watermelon to round out this meal.

MAKES 4 SERVINGS

½ pound lean ground beef
1 tablespoon Worcestershire sauce
1 tablespoon dried minced onion
4 ounces blue cheese crumbles, about ½ cup
4 sesame seed rolls, halved
4 teaspoons olive oil
1 teaspoon garlic powder
1 cup baby spinach
4 slices tomato
2 cups cubed watermelon

1. Preheat the broiler. Heat a George Foreman–type grill to medium-high.

2. Mix the beef with Worcestershire sauce and onion in a large bowl. Form into four balls.

3. Using your fingers, make an indent in each ball and press 1 ounce of blue cheese into the meat. Form meat around the cheese and flatten into a patty.

4. Place the burgers on the bottom of the grill, close the top, and cook until no pink remains, 5 to 6 minutes.

5. Meanwhile, brush the rolls with olive oil, sprinkle with garlic powder, and toast under the broiler, 1 minute.

6. Place ¼ cup of spinach and one slice of the tomato on half of the roll. Top with a burger and other half of roll.

7. Serve each person one burger with ½ cup of watermelon.

Chapter 11
SALADS

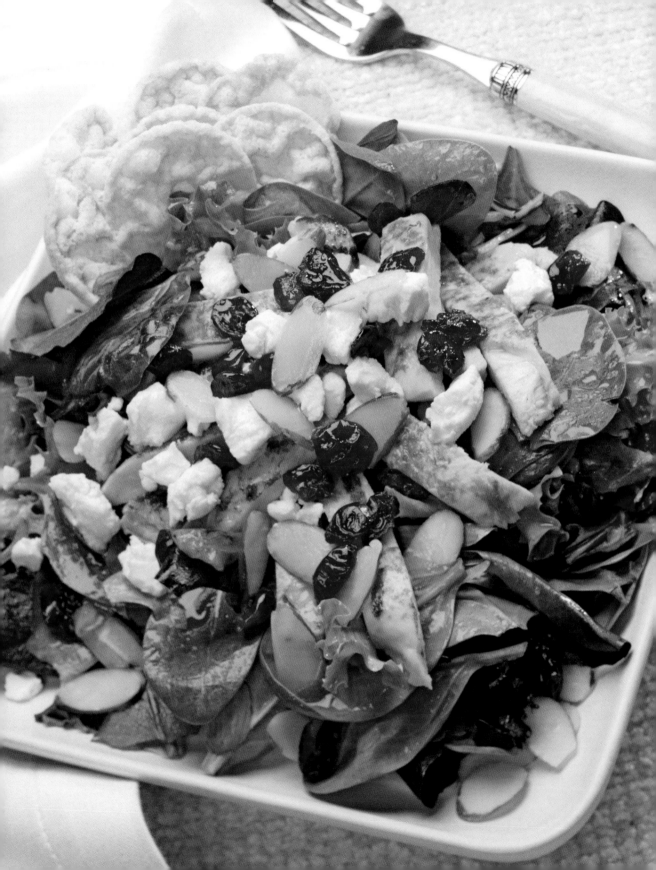

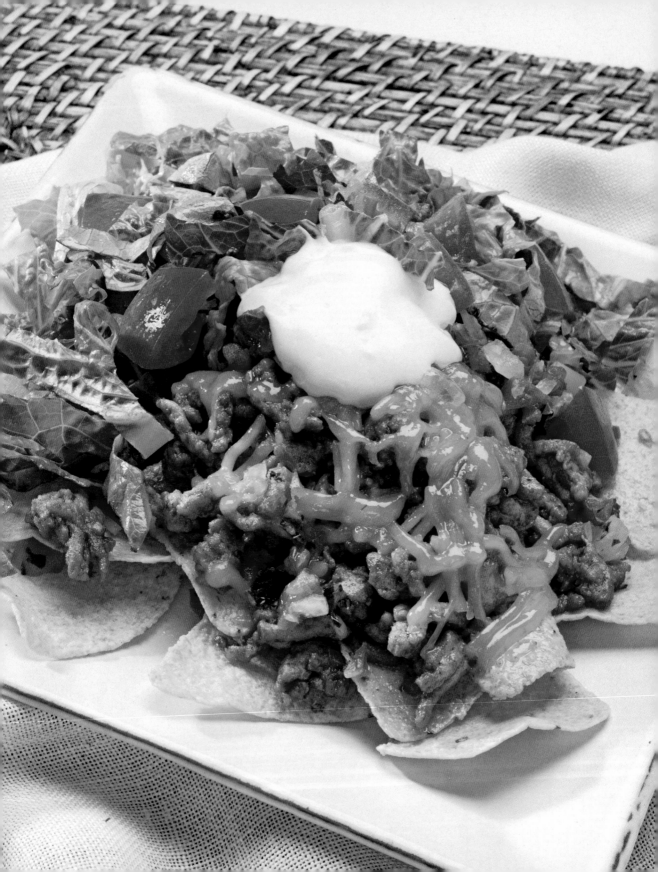

TACO SALAD

Taco salad is typically thought of as the most fattening, unhealthy salad you can order. However, using ground turkey instead of beef, baked tortilla chips, and low-fat sour cream while exercising a little portion control puts this Mexican favorite back on the menu.

MAKES 4 SERVINGS

½ pound ground turkey
½ taco seasoning packet
4 ounces baked tortilla chips
4 ounces shredded cheddar, about ½ cup
2 cups shredded romaine lettuce
2 cups chopped tomato
3 tablespoons low-fat sour cream
1 cup prepared salsa

1. Heat a large nonstick skillet over medium heat.

2. Add the turkey and taco seasoning to the skillet and brown until no pink remains. Drain off the fat.

3. Spread the tortilla chips evenly on four plates.

4. Divide the ground turkey over the chips on each plate and sprinkle evenly with the shredded cheddar.

5. Microwave on low until the cheddar just starts to melt, about 1 mintue.

6. Top each plate with ½ a cup lettuce, ½ a cup chopped tomato, ¾ tablespoon sour cream, and ¼ cup salsa. Serve.

CHICKEN AND CRANBERRY SALAD

Cranberries not only taste delicious, but they also help fight urinary tract infections. Cranberries reduce the ability for *E. coli* bacteria to adhere to the lining of the urinary wall, which helps prevent infection.

MAKES 4 SERVINGS

Cooking spray
1 pound chicken breast tenders
Salt and freshly ground black pepper
8 cups mixed salad greens
4 ounces goat cheese, about ½ cup
½ cup whole almonds
½ cup dried cranberries
3 tablespoons balsamic vinaigrette
4 ounces Genisoy® Soy Crisps

1. Heat a grill pan or George Foreman type–grill to medium-high and spray with cooking spray.

2. Season the chicken tenders with salt and freshly ground black pepper.

3. Grill the chicken until cooked through and no longer pink in the middle, 5 minutes per side. Cool and cut into bite-size pieces.

4. Place the salad greens in a large mixing bowl. Add the cheese, almonds, cranberries, and chicken and toss with the dressing. Divide evenly among four plates.

5. Serve each person one salad with ¼ ounce Genisoy® crisps on the side.

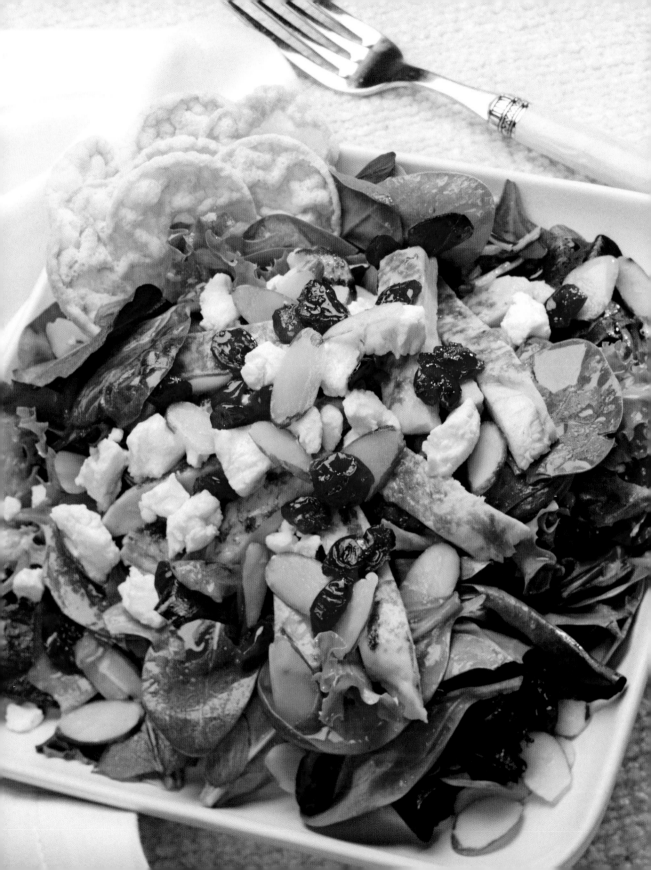

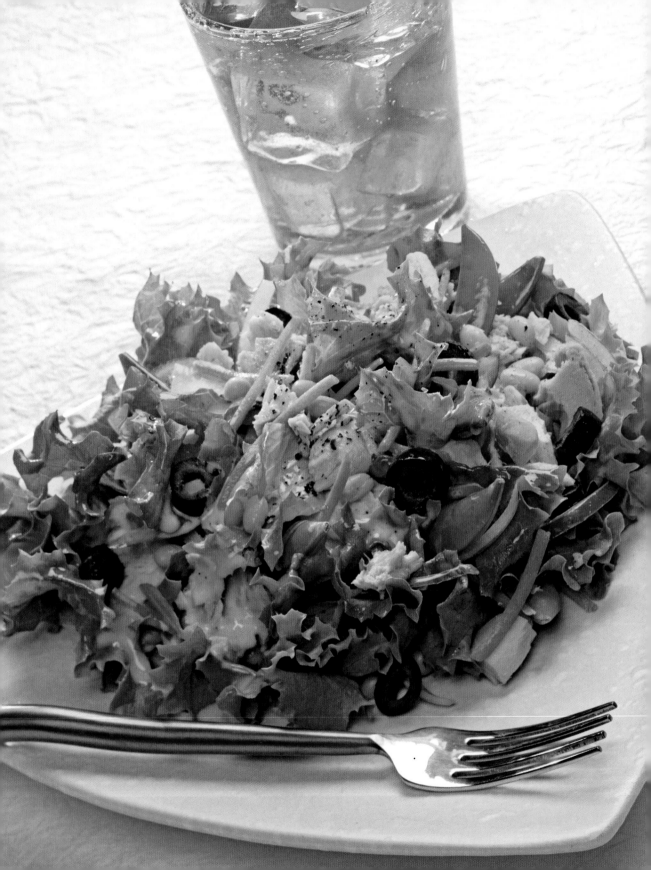

TUNA, BEAN, AND VEGETABLE SALAD

Small white beans, such as navy beans, pack the protein into this hearty tuna salad. Beans are high in starch, protein, and dietary fiber and are an excellent source of iron and folic acid.

MAKES 4 SERVINGS

One 6-ounce pouch or can water-packed tuna, drained
One 15-ounce can small white beans, rinsed and drained
1 cup sugar snap peas
1 cup shredded carrots
½ cup chopped red onion, about ½ medium
4 cups mixed salad greens
¾ cup fat-free ranch dressing
2 tablespoons canned sliced black olives, drained

1. Mix tuna, beans, sugar snaps, carrots, onion, and salad greens in a large bowl.

2. Toss with salad dressing and divide equally among four plates.

3. Top each with ½ tablespoon black olives and serve.

SPINACH BEET SALAD

Enjoy a grilled chicken breast with this gorgeous, magenta beet and spinach salad. Beets, which contain significant amounts of vitamin C, are also high in dietary fiber and several antioxidants.

MAKES 4 SERVINGS

Cooking spray
1 pound chicken breast tenders
Salt and fresh ground black pepper
6 cups baby spinach
Two 15-ounce cans sliced beets, rinsed and drained
¼ cup pepitas (toasted pumpkin seeds)
½ cup diced red onion, about ½ medium
4 ounces feta, about ½ cup
4 tablespoons balsamic vinaigrette

1. Heat a grill pan or George Foreman type–grill to medium-high and spray with cooking spray.

2. Season the chicken with salt and pepper and place on the bottom of the grill and close the top. Grill until cooked through and no longer pink in the middle, 5 minutes per side.

3. Combine the spinach, beets, pepitas, onion, feta, and dressing in a large bowl. Toss to coat. Divide evenly among four salad plates.

4. Serve each person one-fourth of the chicken and one salad.

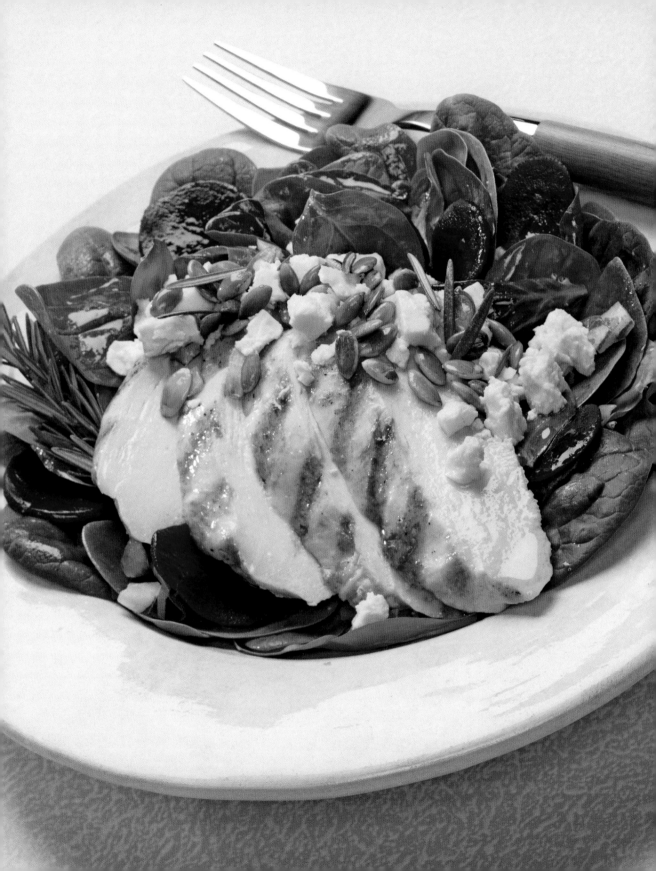

SALMON SALAD

You can use canned salmon or salmon left over from another meal to make this delicious and quick salad.

MAKES 4 SERVINGS

8 cups mixed salad greens
12 ounces cooked salmon (canned in water, drained, is okay)
½ cup grated Parmesan cheese
2 small red bell peppers, sliced into strips
¼ medium seedless cucumber, sliced
3 tablespoons prepared vinaigrette
4 medium pears

1. Combine the salad greens, salmon, Parmesan, bell peppers, cucumber, and dressing. Toss to coat in a large bowl. Divide evenly among four salad plates.

2. Serve each person one salad with one pear on the side.

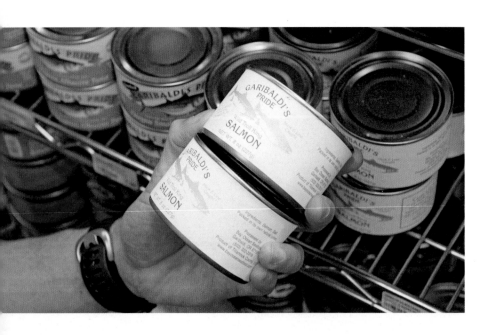

CRABMEAT SALAD PLATE

Crab and other shellfish are excellent sources of lean protein. Shellfish is a good source of chromium, which helps regulate blood glucose levels. Studies have also found that shellfish help raise HDL (good cholesterol) levels, so it helps reduce the risk for coronary artery disease and stroke.

MAKES 4 SERVINGS

Cooking spray
Two 6-inch pita breads, each cut into 6 triangles
½ teaspoon seasoned salt
¾ pound lump crabmeat
2 green onions, chopped
2 tablespoons chopped pimiento
½ cup fat-free blue cheese dressing
4 cups mixed salad greens
2 cups baby carrots
2 cups grape tomatoes

1. Preheat the oven to 400°F. Spray the pita with nonstick cooking spray and sprinkle with ¼ teaspoon of the seasoned salt. Place on a cookie sheet in a hot oven until browned and crisp, 8 minutes.

2. Gently fold together the crabmeat, the remaining seasoned salt, onions, pimiento, and dressing.

3. Divide the salad greens equally among four plates. Evenly distribute carrots, tomatoes, and crabmeat mixture on top of the salad greens.

4. Serve each person one salad with three pita triangles.

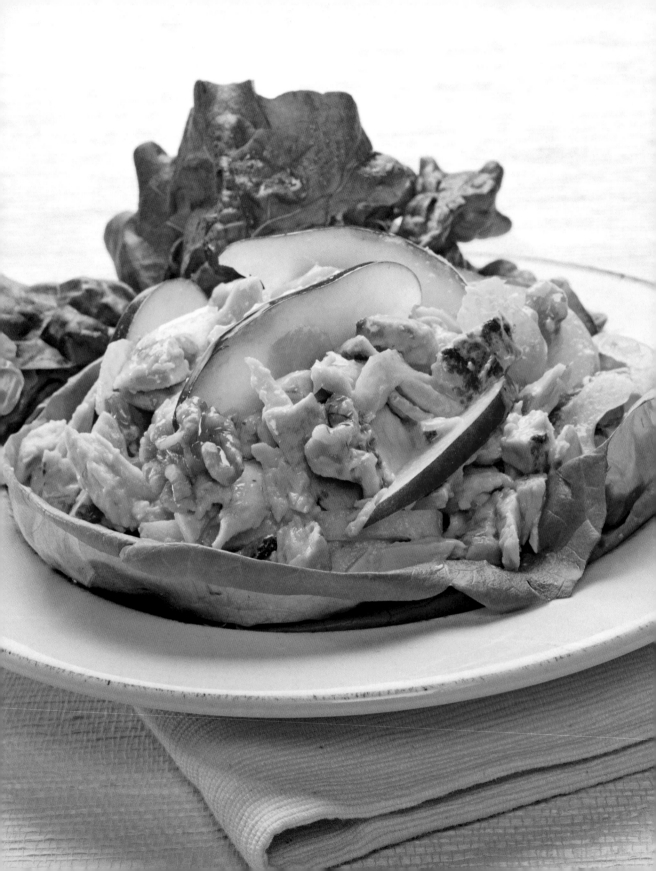

CHICKEN WALDORF SALAD

We've lightened this rich salad, traditionally made with mayonnaise and sour cream, by substituting plain yogurt in place of mayonnaise. Use leftover chicken or cook from scratch to make this lovely salad.

Makes 4 servings

½ cup plain yogurt
2 tablespoons lemon juice, about 1 lemon
½ teaspoon salt
¼ teaspoon freshly ground black pepper
12 ounces cooked chicken breast meat, shredded
2 apples, thinly sliced
3 celery stalks, thinly sliced
¼ cup walnut pieces
4 cups mixed salad greens

1. In a large bowl, whisk together the yogurt, lemon juice, salt, and pepper.

2. Add the chicken, apples, celery, and walnuts to the yogurt mixture and toss to coat.

3. Line four salad plates with salad greens. Divide the chicken mixture evenly among the four plates and serve.

GRILLED SHRIMP CAESAR SALAD

Typically Caesar salad is high in fat and low in nutrition. Grilled shrimp and light dressing make this Caesar a diet-friendly favorite.

MAKES 4 SERVINGS

1 pound shelled, deveined shrimp, tails removed
½ cup fat-free vinaigrette
2 tablespoons minced garlic
Two 10-ounce packages low-fat Caesar salad mix with dressing
2 cups cherry tomatoes
2 tablespoons dill, chopped
4 small whole grain rolls

1. Heat a grill pan or George Foreman–type grill to high.

2. Mix the shrimp with the vinaigrette and garlic in a small bowl. Add the shrimp to the grill and cook until opaque, 2 minutes per side.

3. Toss the salad mix and dressing with the tomatoes, dill, and shrimp in a large bowl.

4. Divide evenly among four salad plates and serve with a whole grain roll.

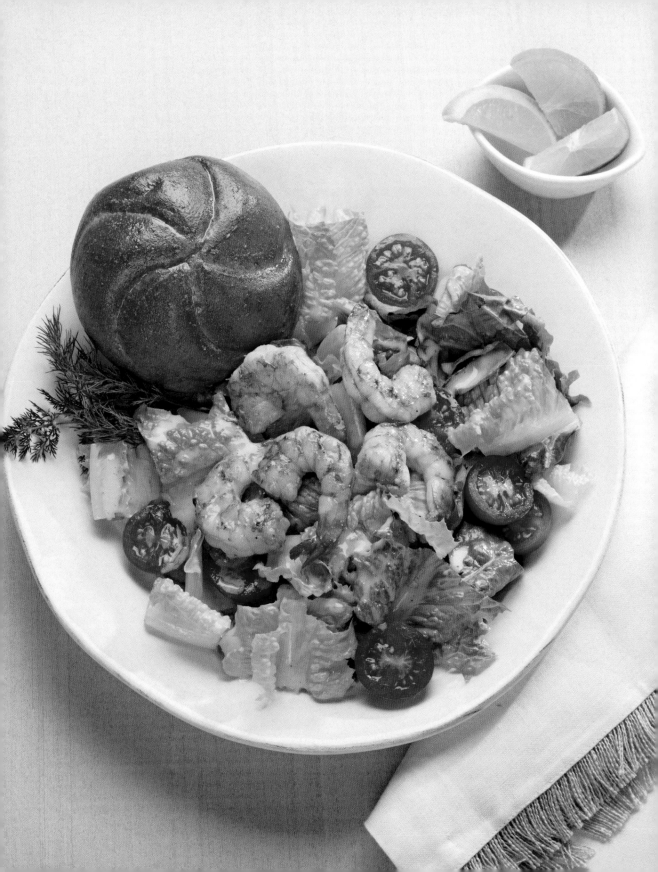

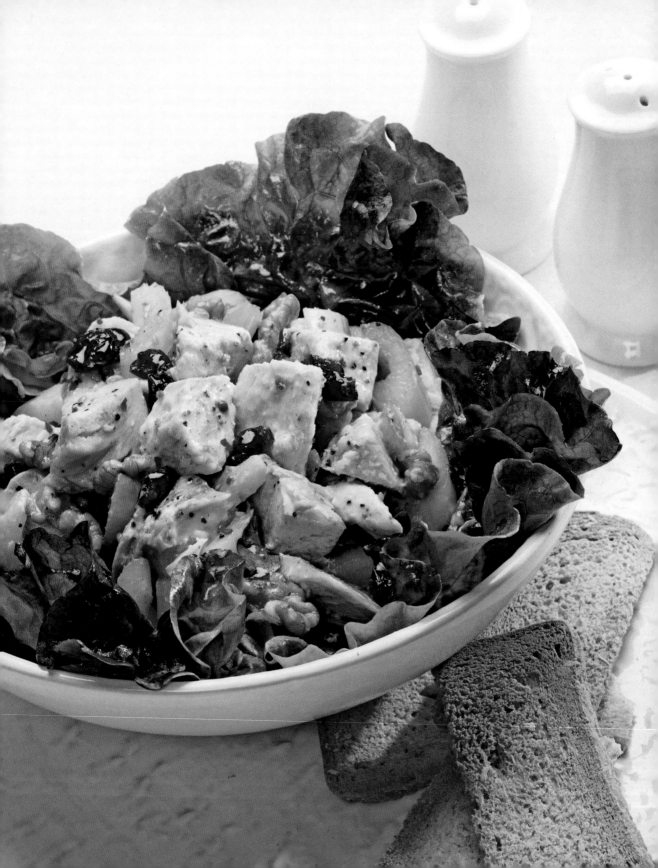

CHUNKY TURKEY SALAD WITH CRANBERRIES AND WALNUTS

Walnuts make this chunky turkey and cranberry salad an essential fatty acid winner. Certain fatty acids are classified as essential because they cannot be synthesized in the body—they must be obtained from food.

MAKES 4 SERVINGS

2 tablespoons chopped walnuts
¾ pound oven-roasted turkey breast, thickly sliced (deli turkey is okay)
½ cup fat-free salad dressing-type mayonnaise, such as Miracle Whip®
1 tablespoon lemon juice
1 tablespoon grill seasoning
¼ cup dried cranberries
1 cup chopped celery
4 cups mixed salad greens
16 slices melba toast

1. Preheat the oven to 400°F.

2. Place the walnuts on a cookie sheet and bake until they smell fragrant, 5 minutes.

3. Dice the turkey into ½-inch cubes.

4. Mix the salad dressing, lemon juice, and grill seasoning in a small bowl. Toss with the turkey cubes, cranberries, and celery.

5. Place one cup of salad greens on each of four plates.

6. Divide the turkey mixture evenly among the four plates. Sprinkle with the toasted walnuts and serve each person one salad with four slices of melba toast.

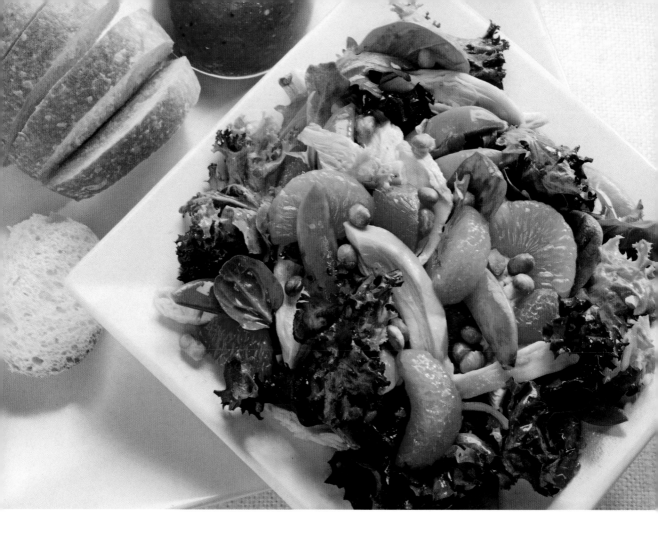

CITRUS CHICKEN SALAD

This tangy chicken salad is made crunchy with soy nuts. Soy nuts are a veggie alternative to bacon bits and add a salty flavor to any salad.

MAKES 4 SERVINGS

12 ounces cooked chicken breast meat, diced
8 cups mixed salad greens
2 cups of juice-packed grapefruit and/or orange sections, drained
1 cup snow peas
½ cup soy nuts
½ cup low-fat Italian dressing
4 small sourdough rolls

1. Combine the chicken, salad greens, grapefruit and/or orange segments, snow peas, and soy nuts and toss with the dressing in a large bowl.

2. Divide evenly among four plates and serve each person one salad with one roll.

SPINACH SALAD

This spinach salad provides vitamins A and K, fiber, and antioxidants from the spinach; protein from the eggs and cheese; and beta-carotene from the carrots. Enjoy this healthy take on traditional, bacon-dressed spinach salad without one ounce of the guilt!

MAKES 4 SERVINGS

4 slices bacon
8 cups baby spinach
4 hard-boiled eggs, peeled and quartered lengthwise
2 ounces Swiss cheese, cut into 1-inch pieces, about ¼ cup
2 tablespoons Parmesan
1 cup cherry tomatoes
1 cup shredded carrots
1 cucumber, peeled and sliced
4 tablespoons low-fat Italian dressing
4 small whole grain rolls

1. Cook the bacon in the microwave according to the package instructions. Drain and cut into 1-inch pieces.

2. Combine the bacon, spinach, eggs, cheeses, tomatoes, carrots, and cucumber and toss with the dressing in a large bowl.

3. Divide equally among four plates and serve each person one salad with one roll.

Chapter 12
VEGETARIAN

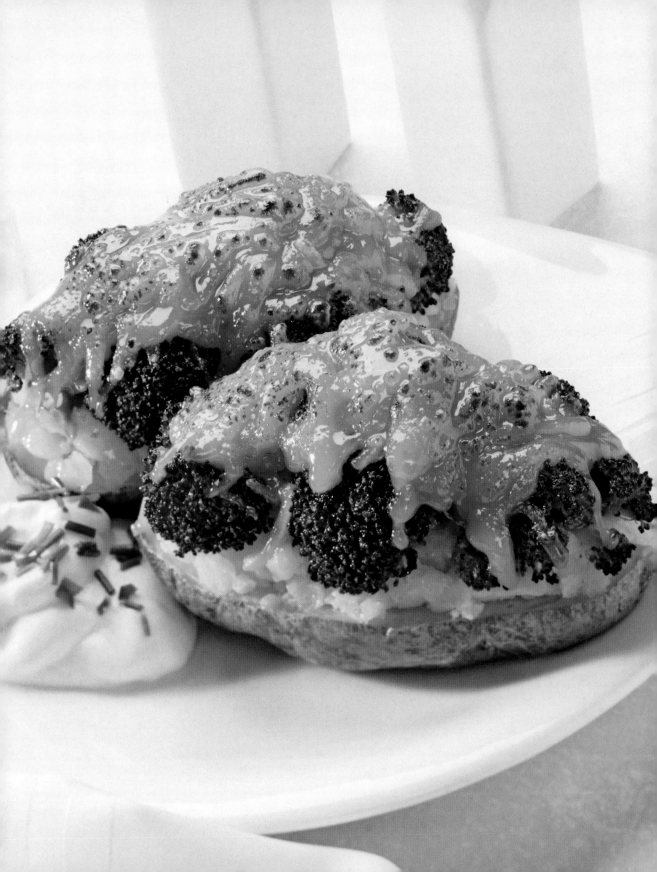

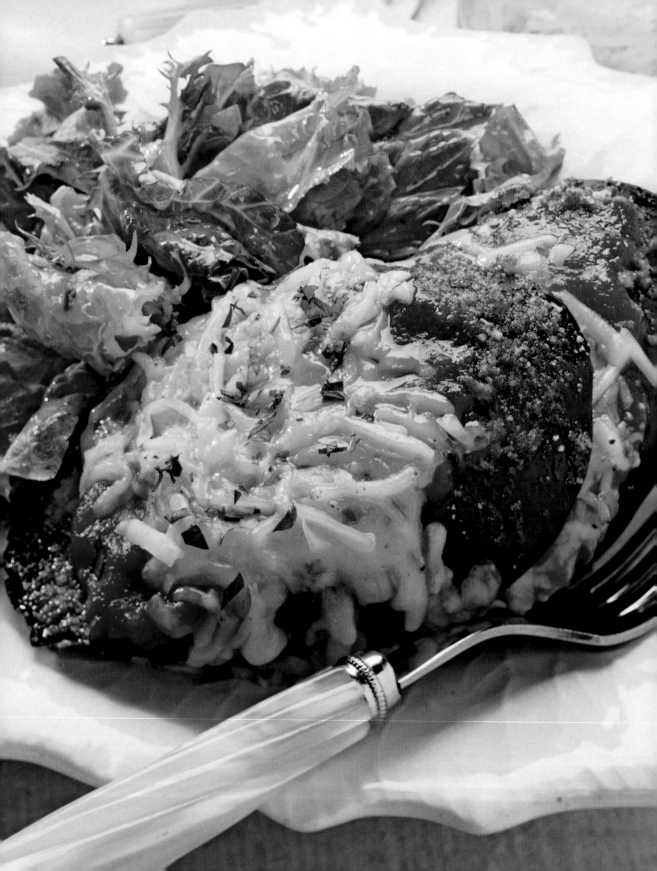

GRILLED EGGPLANT PARMESAN

Typically, eggplant Parmesan includes breaded, fried eggplant smothered with tons of full-fat cheese. Our version uses grilled eggplant and low-fat cheese to lighten this vegetarian favorite.

MAKES 4 SERVINGS

Cooking spray
3 teaspoons olive oil
2 teaspoons garlic powder
1 large eggplant, sliced lengthwise into 1-inch slices
6 tablespoons seasoned bread crumbs
2 cups prepared marinara sauce
10 ounces shredded part-skim mozzarella cheese, about 1¼ cups
2 ounces grated Parmesan
4 cups mixed salad greens
¼ cup fat-free Italian dressing

1. Preheat a grill or grill pan over medium-high heat and spray with cooking spray. Preheat the broiler. Line a baking sheet with aluminum foil.

2. Combine the oil, garlic powder, and eggplant in a large zip-top bag and shake to coat the eggplant.

3. Place the eggplant on the grill and cook on both sides until softened, 2 minutes per side.

4. Remove the eggplant from the grill and coat with bread crumbs. Place on the baking sheet and put under the broiler until bread crumbs brown, 1 minute. Turn the eggplant and broil the other side until brown, 1 minute more.

5. Remove from the broiler, and top with the marinara sauce and cheeses.

6.   Put the eggplant back under the broiler and heat until the sauce warms and the cheese melts, 2 to 3 minutes.

7.   Meanwhile, toss the salad greens with the dressing in a large bowl and divide evenly among four plates.

8.   Serve each person one-fourth of the eggplant Parmesan with one salad.

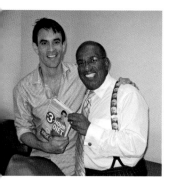

VEGETARIAN CHILI

I created this recipe for my good friend and client Al Roker—based on his family's old-style chili. My goal was to create a chili that tasted delicious, was filling, and had zero guilt. He and I cooked this together on the *Today Show*. It was a smashing success!

MAKES 4 SERVINGS

Three 15-ounce cans Health Valley® Vegetarian Chili
2 large onions, diced
6 garlic cloves, chopped
1 tablespoon paprika
1 tablespoon chili powder
One 32-ounce can crushed tomatoes
4 ounces shredded cheddar cheese, about ½ cup
4 medium oranges

1.   Heat a medium saucepan over medium heat.

2.   Combine the chili, onions, garlic, paprika, chili powder, and tomatoes in the saucepan and bring to a boil. Reduce heat and simmer the chili, uncovered, 8 minutes.

3.   Divide the chili evenly among four bowls and top with cheddar cheese. Serve each person one bowl of chili with one orange.

GARDENBURGERS WITH VEGETABLE CRUDITÉS

Creating crudites sounds like a complicated process, but it's really just chopping small pieces of raw vegetables, such as carrots and red peppers, to be eaten as an appetizer or snack. Serve these crudites with a Gardenburger and sweet potato coins.

MAKES 4 SERVINGS

Cooking spray
4 Gardenburger frozen vegetarian burgers
2 medium sweet potatoes, sliced into ½-inch coin-shaped pieces
Salt and freshly ground black pepper
8 slices whole grain bread
4 tablespoons mustard
4 tablespoons fat-free mayonnaise
1 cup mixed greens
2 cups baby carrots
2 cups sliced red bell pepper

1. Heat a grill or grill pan to medium-high and spray with cooking spray.

2. Place the Gardenburgers and sweet potato coins on the grill and cook until crispy, about 10 minutes, turning once halfway through cooking.

3. Sprinkle the sweet potato coins with salt and pepper to taste.

4. Toast the bread and spread with the mustard and mayonnaise. Top four slices of the bread with ¼ cup of greens. Add one Gardenburger patty to each and top with the remaining slices of bread.

5. Serve each person one Gardenburger, one-fourth of the sweet potato coins, ½ cup carrots, and ½ cup bell pepper slices.

BURRITO AND GREENS

Amy's burritos are organic, low-fat, and taste great. This quick and easy meal is great for vegetarians on the run.

MAKES 4 SERVINGS

4 Amy's® frozen Bean and Cheese Burritos
4 cups mixed salad greens
½ large cucumber, chopped
1 large tomato, chopped
3 tablespoons vinaigrette

1. Microwave the burritos according to the package instructions.

2. Combine the salad greens, cucumber, tomato, and vinaigrette and toss to coat in a large mixing bowl. Divide equally among four salad plates.

3. Serve each person one burrito with one salad.

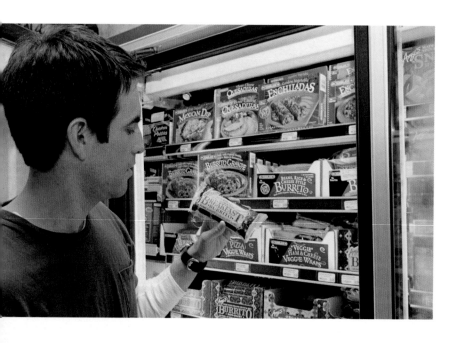

BEAN BURRITO

Our unique take on a bean burrito incorporates red kidney beans with the traditional refried beans to bulk up this vegetarian standby.

MAKES 4 SERVINGS

½ cup fat-free refried beans
Four 6-inch flour tortillas
One 15-ounce can red kidney beans, rinsed and drained
10 ounces reduced-fat shredded cheddar cheese, about 1¼ cups
2 cups mixed salad greens
2 cups chopped fresh tomatoes
½ cup reduced-fat salad dressing

1. Preheat the oven to 475°F.

2. Spread 2 tablespoons of the refried beans over each tortilla. Place ½ cup kidney beans in the center of each tortilla. Sprinkle the cheese evenly over each tortilla. Roll the tortilla tightly to enclose the filling and place seam side down in a small baking dish. Bake until the cheese melts, 5 minutes.

3. Toss the salad greens and tomatoes with the salad dressing in a large bowl and divide evenly among four plates.

4. Serve each person one burrito with one salad.

POTATO STUFFED WITH BROCCOLI AND MELTED CHEDDAR

For baked potato lovers, this meal is a real treat. Stuffed with steamed broccoli and creamy cheddar cheese, these potatoes taste as good as they look.

MAKES 4 SERVINGS

4 small russet potatoes
10 ounces broccoli florets
12 ounces shredded low-fat cheddar cheese, about 1½ cups
¾ cup low-fat sour cream
2 tablespoons chopped chives

1. Pierce the potatoes and microwave on high until tender, 6 to 8 minutes.

2. Meanwhile, place the broccoli in a large saucepan with 3 tablespoons water over medium heat. Cover and cook for 6 to 7 minutes or until tender. Drain and return the broccoli to the pan.

3. Add the cheddar cheese to the broccoli and stir over low heat until the cheese is melted.

4. Slice the potatoes lengthwise and divide the cheese-broccoli sauce evenly over each potato. Top each potato with 3 tablespoons of sour cream.

5. Serve each person two potato halves garnished with chives.

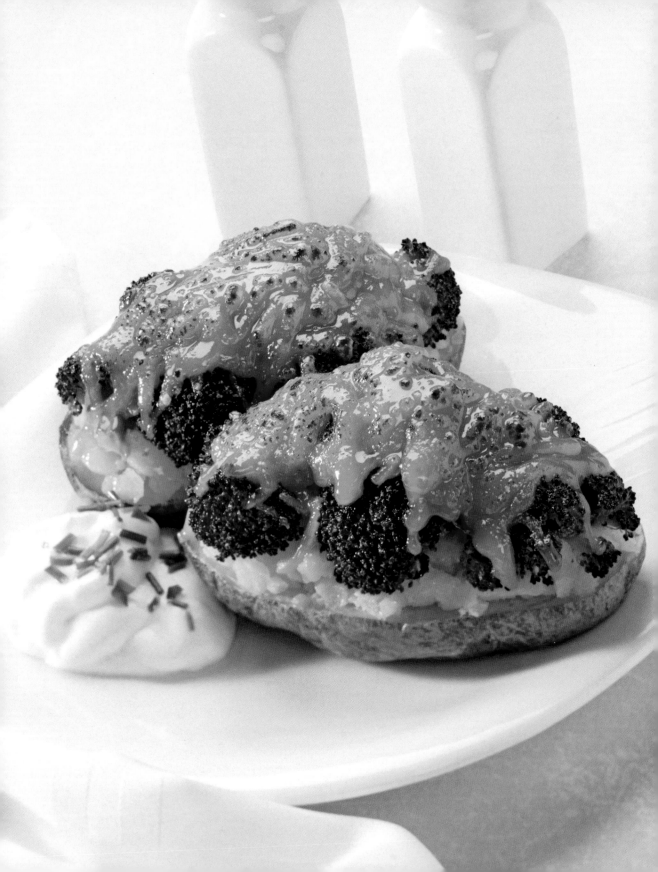

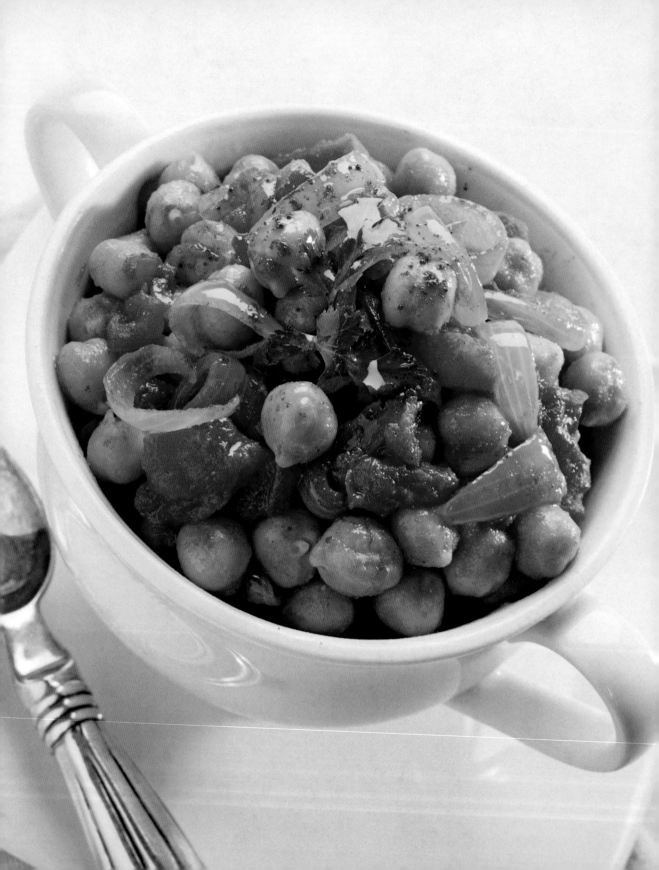

CHICKPEA VEGETABLE CURRY

Chickpeas, or garbanzo beans, are an excellent source of high-quality, low-fat protein. They're also a perfect choice for people with diabetes, insulin resistance, and hypoglycemia because they prevent blood sugar levels from rising too rapidly after a meal. Moreover, chickpeas contain a lot of fiber, which makes you feel full so you don't overeat.

MAKES 4 SERVINGS

1 tablespoon olive oil
½ medium yellow onion, thinly sliced
½ to 1 tablespoon curry powder, to taste
½ to 1 teaspoon salt, to taste
½ teaspoon turmeric
2 tablespoons minced garlic
One 14.5-ounce can diced tomatoes (fire-roasted if available)
1 can chickpeas, rinsed and drained
2 tablespoons chopped fresh cilantro

1. Heat a large nonstick skillet over medium heat and add the oil.

2. Add the onion, curry powder, salt (begin with ½ teaspoon each of the salt and curry, and adjust seasonings after the remaining ingredients are incorporated), turmeric, and garlic to the skillet.

3. Sauté, stirring often, until the onion begins to soften, 5 minutes. Add the tomatoes and chickpeas.

4. Bring the mixture to a boil and reduce heat to low. Simmer for 8 minutes.

5. Divide the mixture among four plates, garnish with cilantro, and serve.

FRANKS AND BEANS

Tofu Pups are a delicious, meatless alternative to the traditional hot dog. These pups can be boiled or grilled, so don't hesitate to bring them to the spring picnic.

MAKES 4 SERVINGS

Two 15-ounce cans Eden® baked beans
4 tofu hot dogs (Tofu Pups®)
4 whole grain hot dog buns
Prepared mustard to taste
1 seedless cucumber, sliced
2 green bell peppers, sliced

1. Put the baked beans into a medium saucepan over medium heat and bring to a simmer.

2. Microwave the hot dogs until hot in the middle, about 1 minute.

3. Slather the buns with mustard to taste.

4. Put the hot dogs in the buns and top with the baked beans.

5. Serve each person one hot dog with one-fourth of the cucumber and one-fourth of green pepper slices.

GRILLED HAWAIIAN SOY BURGER

There are many different kinds of soy burgers on the market, and nearly everyone can find a brand they like. Experiment with different brands until you find one that suits your palate.

MAKES 4 SERVINGS

Cooking spray
10 ounces broccoli florets
4 soy-based veggie burgers
4 slices pineapple (thawed if frozen, drained if canned)
2 tablespoons low-fat mayonnaise
2 teaspoons teriyaki sauce
4 whole grain sandwich buns
4 romaine lettuce leaves

1. Heat a grill or grill pan over medium heat and spray with cooking spray.

2. Bring 2 inches of water to a simmer in a large stockpot and place a steamer basket in the pot. Add the broccoli and cover. Steam until tender, 6 minutes.

3. Put the veggie burgers and pineapple on the grill. Cook until browned and heated through, 3 to 4 minutes per side.

4. Stir together the mayonnaise and teriyaki sauce in a small bowl. Divide and spread evenly on buns. Add one soy burger, lettuce, and pineapple to each bun and top with bun top.

5. Serve each person one burger with one-fourth of the broccoli.

SOY CRUMBLE PITAS

Soy crumbles and mozzarella cheese pack the protein into this veggie sandwich, while the bell pepper provides plenty of vitamin C. Whole grain pitas fill you up, and a sweet pear rounds out this simple meal.

MAKES 4 SERVINGS

1 tablespoon olive oil
8 ounces soy crumbles
½ medium onion, diced
1 medium green bell pepper, diced
½ teaspoon salt
¼ teaspoon freshly ground black pepper
4 ounces shredded skim mozzarella cheese, about ½ cup
2 6-inch whole grain pita pocket breads, halved
4 medium pears

1. Heat a large nonstick skillet over medium heat and add the oil.

2. Add the soy crumbles, onion, and bell pepper. Season with salt and black pepper. Sauté until the onion and pepper are tender and the soy crumbles are heated through, 5 minutes.

3. Divide the soy mixture evenly among the four pita halves. Sprinkle each with 2 tablespoons shredded cheese.

4. Serve each person one pita half with one pear.

MISO SOUP WITH SOBA NOODLES

Miso soup is a traditional Japanese dish made of dissolved, softened miso—a dried, fermented soybean paste. Our version of miso soup includes tofu, buckwheat noodles (soba), and vegetables to give it a full-bodied flavor.

MAKES 4 SERVINGS

4 cups soba noodles
12 ounces firm tofu
1 rib celery, sliced
1 carrot, sliced into rounds
2 heads baby bok choy, sliced
6 tablespoons miso
3 cups mango slices (thawed if frozen, drained if canned)

1. Boil 8 cups of water in a large stockpot over high heat. Add the soba noodles and boil until tender, 8 to 10 minutes.

2. When the noodles are almost tender, add the tofu, celery, carrots, and bok choy. Reduce heat to low. Simmer until the vegetables are soft, 5 minutes.

3. Once the vegetables are soft, remove 1 cup of the liquid, place in a small bowl, and mix in the miso.

4. Add the miso mixture back to the stockpot. Bring back to a simmer, but do not boil.

5. Divide the soup equally into bowls, with ¾ cup mango slices on the side.

MEDITERRANEAN PITA

This pita is similar to a falafel sandwich, which includes a fried chickpea patty, sauce, and vegetables. We've replaced the fried patty with hummus, which has the same health benefits of the fried patty without the excess fat.

MAKES 4 SERVINGS

1 cup hummus
Four 6-inch whole grain pita pocket breads, halved
1 cup mixed salad greens
16 slices tomato
16 slices seedless cucumber
4 ounces crumbled feta cheese, about ½ cup
4 cups grapes

1.   Spread 2 tablespoons of hummus inside each pita pocket half.

2.   Stuff the pita pockets equally with salad greens, tomato, cucumber, and feta.

3.   Serve each person two pita halves with 1 cup of grapes.

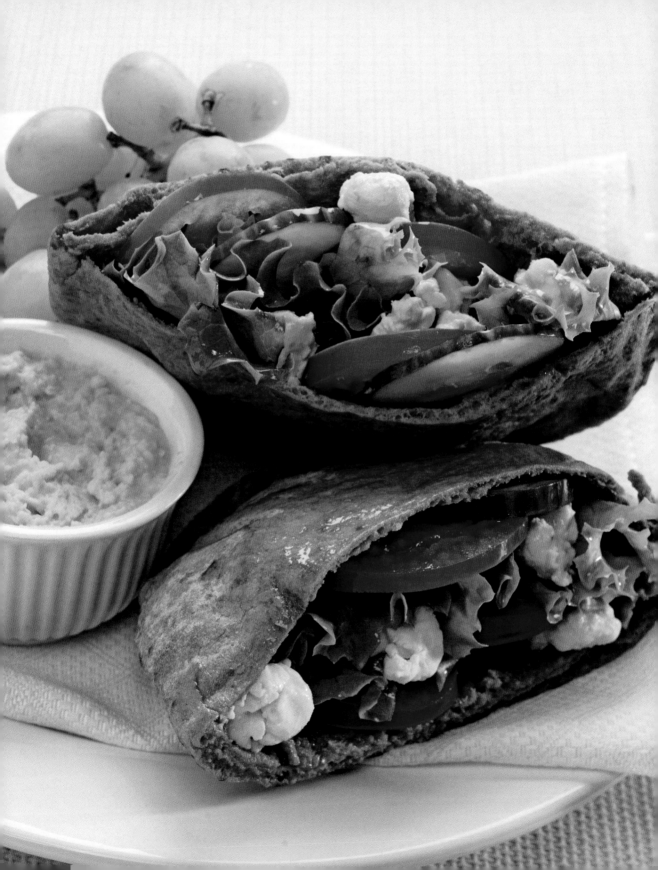

Part 3
MAKING THE MEAL COMPLETE

Chapter 13 SNACKS

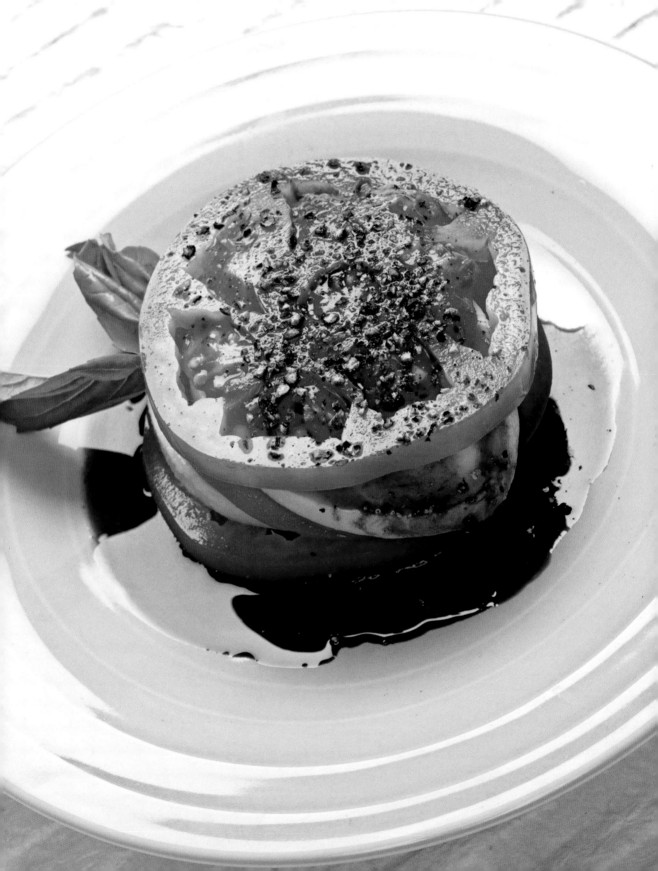

CHOCOLATE-COVERED PRETZELS

Chocolate doesn't just taste delicious, it also has valuable health benefits. Chocolate, and dark chocolate in particular, is rich in antioxidants, which are known to reduce the risk of developing many types of cancer. Antioxidants also help protect you from developing cardiovascular disease. So, enjoy your favorite treat . . . in moderation.

MAKES 1 SERVING

6 pretzel sticks
¼ ounce semisweet chocolate chips

Place the pretzels on a sheet of waxed paper. Put the chocolate chips in a small microwave-safe bowl and microwave until melted, about 15 to 20 seconds, stirring frequently. Drizzle chocolate over pretzels and let it rest until chocolate is firm.

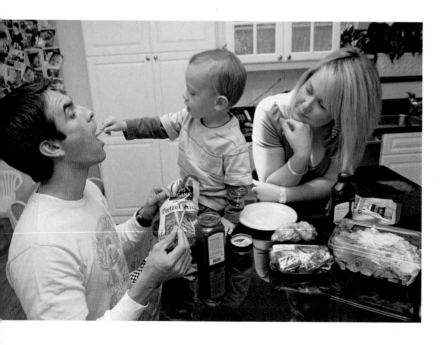

CHEESY POPCORN

Have a yen for a cheesy snack? This delectable popcorn snack will satisfy your craving.

MAKES 1 SERVING

1 snack-size bag of PopSecret® popcorn
½ slice 2% American cheese, diced into ½-inch pieces

Microwave the popcorn according to the package instructions and pour into a large glass bowl. Top the popcorn with diced cheese and microwave for 10 to 15 seconds more or until the cheese is melted.

CEREAL TRAIL MIX

Trail mix is a popular road-trip food because it travels so well. Try this mix in place of your favorite trail mix for your next trip.

MAKES 1 SERVING

½ cup air-popped popcorn
¼ cup Cheerios®
¼ ounce mini pretzels
10 goldfish crackers

Combine all the ingredients in a small bowl and serve.

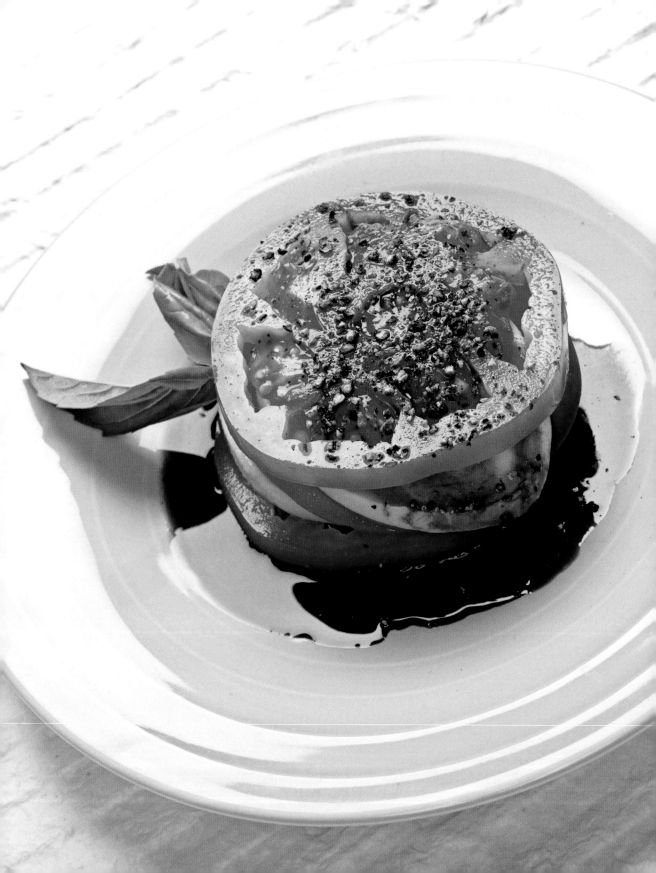

MOZZARELLA AND TOMATO SALAD

This salad, known as Caprese in Italy, makes a beautiful presentation with a fresh basil garnish.

MAKES 1 SERVING

1 ounce part-skim mozzarella cheese, thinly sliced
½ large tomato, thinly sliced
1 medium basil leaf
½ tablespoon balsamic vinegar

Layer the mozzarella and tomato slices on a platter. Garnish with basil and drizzle with balsamic vinegar. Serve.

THREE-BEAN SALAD

For you protein lovers, this three-bean salad is right up your alley. Make it the night before and enjoy it as an afternoon snack at work.

MAKES 1 SERVING

1 tablespoon low-fat Italian salad dressing
½ teaspoon sugar
2 ounces red kidney beans, rinsed and drained
2 ounces canned cut green beans, rinsed and drained
2 ounces canned cut wax beans, rinsed and drained
1 tablespoon chopped onion

In a small bowl, whisk the salad dressing with the sugar until dissolved. Add the beans and onions and toss to coat. Serve.

MINI QUESADILLA

For those afternoons when you have a craving for Mexican food, try one of these cheesy quesadillas. It's sure to put an end to your hunger.

MAKES 1 SERVING

½ ounce shredded low-fat cheddar cheese
¼ scallion, sliced
½ 6-inch flour tortilla
1 tablespoon salsa

1. Heat a nonstick skillet over medium heat.

2. Place the cheese and scallion on the tortilla and fold in half. Take care not to put filling too close to the edges or it may leak during heating.

3. Add the quesadilla to the skillet and heat until the cheese melts, flipping halfway through the cooking time, 4 minutes per side.

4. Serve with salsa.

APPLE AND PEANUT BUTTER

Apples and peanut butter make a delicious and satisfying combination of sweet and savory. The peanut butter satiates your appetite while the apple satisfies your sweet tooth.

MAKES 1 SERVING

½ medium apple, sliced
⅛ teaspoon cinnamon
1 tablespoon creamy peanut butter

Sprinkle apple slices with cinnamon. Serve with peanut butter for dipping.

COTTAGE CHEESE AND FRUIT

Light, refreshing melon pairs beautifully with rich, creamy cottage cheese. Garnish the plate with red leaf lettuce if you can find it; the pretty presentation will heighten your enjoyment of this simple snack.

MAKES 1 SERVING

1 large lettuce leaf
½ cup 1% cottage cheese
½ cup mixed melon cubes

Place the lettuce leaf on a plate. Place a mound of cottage cheese in the center of the plate. Surround with melon and serve.

OPEN-FACED CHEESE MELT

Light bread and fat-free American cheese make it possible to enjoy this mouthwatering open-faced cheese melt whenever you desire.

MAKES 1 SERVING

1 slice reduced-calorie whole grain bread
1 slice tomato
1 slice fat-free American cheese

1.　Preheat the broiler.

2.   Lightly toast the bread under the broiler, 2 minutes.

3.   Put tomato and cheese on the toast.

4.   Place open-faced sandwich under the broiler and heat until the cheese melts, 2 minutes. Serve.

RICOTTA AND BERRY PARFAIT

Naturally low-fat ricotta cheese has a slight sweetness to it, which makes it well-suited to fruit pairings. Look for berries in season; they'll be much sweeter and more affordable than berries out of season.

MAKES 1 SERVING

¼ cup part-skim ricotta cheese
½ packet artificial sweetener
½ cup mixed berries (thawed if frozen)
½ tablespoon nonfat whipped topping
¼ teaspoon cinnamon

Mix the ricotta with the sweetener and layer with the berries in a clear glass. Top with the whipped topping, sprinkle with cinnamon, and serve.

TURKEY AND APPLESAUCE HALF SANDWICH

The applesauce spread on this sandwich makes it taste like dessert, while the turkey gives you sustenance to get through a long afternoon at work.

MAKES 1 SERVING

1 slice reduced-calorie bread
1 teaspoon applesauce
1 thin slice deli-style turkey
1 leaf lettuce

Spread the applesauce on the bread. Add the turkey and lettuce. Fold the sandwich in half and serve.

BLUE CHEESE RICE CAKE

If you're in the mood for something crunchy, rice cakes are a terrific alternative to chips. Low in fat and calories, they gratify you when you need a snack.

MAKES 1 SERVING

1 rice cake
1 tablespoon fat-free sour cream
1 tablespoon crumbled blue cheese

Spread the sour cream on the rice cake. Sprinkle with the blue cheese and serve.

PEANUT BUTTER RASPBERRY HALF SANDWICH

If you're hungry, you can't go wrong with peanut butter. It's filling, healthy, and provides high-quality protein.

MAKES 1 SERVING

½ tablespoon peanut butter
1 slice reduced-calorie bread
1 tablespoon fat-free raspberry vinaigrette dressing

Spread the peanut butter on the bread. Sprinkle vinaigrette onto the peanut butter. Fold the bread in half and serve.

COTTAGE CHEESE AND APPLESAUCE HALF SANDWICH

This sweet and savory sandwich satisfies your appetite and your sweet tooth.

MAKES 1 SERVING

¼ cup low-fat cottage cheese
2 tablespoons applesauce
1 slice reduced-calorie bread
¼ teaspoon cinnamon

In a small bowl, combine the cottage cheese and applesauce. Spread the cottage cheese mixture onto the bread. Sprinkle with cinnamon and serve.

PEANUT BUTTER GRAHAM CRACKER

Graham crackers have a hint of sweetness that pairs well with the flavor of peanut butter.

MAKES 1 SERVING

2 graham cracker squares
1 teaspoon peanut butter

Spread the peanut butter onto the graham crackers and serve.

PITA WITH HUMMUS

Try toasting the pita slices for a crunchy variation on this Middle Eastern favorite.

MAKES 1 SERVING

½ 6-inch whole grain pita bread
1 tablespoon hummus

Cut the pita into quarters. Serve with hummus for dipping.

VEGGIES AND DIP

There are many types of fat-free ranch dressings on the shelves of the supermarket. Find the one that you like best and use it as a dip for veggies.

MAKES 1 SERVING

¼ cup fat-free ranch dressing
¼ cup celery sticks
¼ cup carrot sticks
¼ cup cherry tomatoes
¼ cup red bell pepper slices

Dip your vegetable of choice into dressing and enjoy.

GRAHAM CRACKER AND MARSHMALLOW

This healthier variation of s'mores will remind you of childhood campfires without damaging your waistline.

MAKES 1 SERVING

1 large marshmallow
1 graham cracker square
¼ teaspoon Hershey's chocolate syrup

Place the graham cracker on a microwave-safe plate and top with marshmallow. Microwave until gooey, 30 seconds. Drizzle the marshmallow square with chocolate syrup and serve.

GELATIN AND WHIPPED TOPPING

This is a jiggly, fun snack that you can have anytime of day. The whipped topping adds a creamy contrast to the cool gelatin.

MAKES 1 SERVING

½ cup sugar-free prepared gelatin, any flavor, cubed
2 tablespoons low-fat whipped topping

Place the gelatin cubes in a martini glass. Top with whipped topping and serve.

JUICE SORBET

This snack is similar to sorbet but lower in calories. Try it with the fruit juice of your choice.

MAKES 1 SERVING

1 cup orange juice or any low-calorie juice of your choice

Pour the juice into a small baking dish and freeze until solid. Scrape with a fork to form slushy ice crystals. Place the ice in a small cup and serve.

PICKLE WRAP

Sometimes we all have a craving for pickles. Wrap this pickle in ham and cheese for a delectable and quick snack.

MAKES 1 SERVING

1 large dill pickle
1 thin slice deli ham
1 thin slice Swiss cheese

Wrap the ham and Swiss cheese around the pickle and serve.

STUFFED CELERY

Peanut butter and celery take on a new flavor when you add a little soft light cream cheese. Try this the next time you have a craving for a rich snack.

MAKES 1 SERVING

1 tablespoon light cream cheese, softened
1 tablespoon chunky peanut butter
1 large stalk celery

In a small bowl, stir together the cream cheese and peanut butter. Stuff the celery with the peanut butter mixture and serve.

TACO BROCCOLI

This little snack has the taste of Mexico. Enjoy healthy broccoli with a dollop of taco-seasoned sour cream for a creamy, satisfying snack.

MAKES 1 SERVING

¼ cup low-fat sour cream
¾ teaspoon taco seasoning
½ cup broccoli florets

Stir together the sour cream and taco seasoning in a small bowl. Serve the mixture with broccoli florets for dipping.

MINI PIZZA

Triscuit™ pizzas are cute, delicious, and satisfying. Keep these ingredients on hand for a quick and easy snack.

MAKES 1 SERVING

½ tablespoon prepared pizza sauce
1 Triscuit™ cracker
½ tablespoon shredded cheddar

Spread the sauce onto the cracker. Top with the cheese and microwave for about 15 seconds. Serve.

CANTALOUPE COOLER

Cantaloupe is rich in vitamin A and beta-carotene, both of which are important for maintaining vision health. In fact, one research study found that people who ate a diet rich in vitamin A and beta-carotene had a 39 percent reduced risk of developing cataracts. Beta-carotene has also been shown to have cancer-fighting properties.

MAKES 1 SERVING

1 cup cantaloupe cubes
½ ripe banana, sliced
¼ cup nonfat vanilla yogurt
¼ cup orange juice
2 ice cubes, cracked

Combine all the ingredients in a blender. Process until smooth. Pour into a tall glass and serve.

DREAMY ORANGE CREAM

This delicious, healthy shake is reminiscent of childhood 50-50 bars. It's a perfect blend of tart orange juice and creamy yogurt.

MAKES 1 SERVING

¾ cup orange juice
½ cup nonfat vanilla frozen yogurt
1½ teaspoons all-fruit orange marmalade
2 ice cubes, cracked
Mint leaf

Combine the orange juice, frozen yogurt, marmalade, and ice cubes in a blender carafe. Process until smooth. Pour into a glass and garnish with mint leaf.

PEACH SMOOTHIE

The touch of cinnamon married with sweet peaches makes this snack taste like a peach pie in a glass.

MAKES 1 SERVING

½ ripe peach, peeled and sliced, or ½ cup canned peaches in juice
2 teaspoons sugar
½ cup nonfat vanilla ice cream
Pinch of ground cinnamon

Put all ingredients in a blender. Blend until smooth. Pour into a glass and serve.

CARIBBEAN FRUIT FRAPPE

This tropical fruit shake will make you think you're relaxing in the Caribbean.

MAKES 1 SERVING

½ cup pineapple cubes
½ cup mango cubes
½ cup low-fat vanilla ice cream
1 tablespoon lime juice, about 1 lime
½ teaspoon coconut extract

In a blender, puree all the ingredients until smooth. Pour into a glass and serve.

NEED EVEN FASTER 100-CALORIE SNACKS? TRY THESE:

FRESH

Apples, green or red
(1 medium)
Apple juice (1 cup)
Applesauce, unsweetened
(1 cup)
Apricots (8)
Bananas (1)
Bell peppers (1, any color)
Bitter melon (1)
Blackberries (1½ cups)
Blueberries (1½ cups)
Boysenberries (1½ cups)
Broccoli (2 cups)
Cantaloupe (2 cups, cubed)
Casaba melon (2 cups, cubed)
Carrots (2 cups)
Cauliflower (2 cups)
Celery and peanut butter
(3 sticks with 1 teaspoon
peanut butter)
Cherries (24 large)
Clementines (2)
Craisins/dried cranberries
(4 tablespoons)
Cranberries, unsweetened
(2 cups)
Cranberry juice (1 cup)
Dannon DanActive,
any flavor (1)
Dannon Light'n Fit Smoothie,
all flavors (1 bottle)
Dannon Light'n Fit Yogurt, all
flavors (6 ounces)
Dannon Light'n Fit Creamy, all
flavors (6 ounces)
Dates (6)
Earthbound Farm Organic
Snack Pack, Carrots with
Ranch Dip (1)
Figs, dried (2)
Figs, fresh (4)

Fruit cocktail (1 cup)
Grapefruit (1)
Grapefruit juice (1 cup)
Grapes, green or red (24)
Guava (3 small)
Honeydew melon (2 cups,
cubed)
Kiwifruit (2 large)
Knudsen On-the-Go Low-Fat
Cottage Cheese (1)
Mandarin orange (1½ cups)
Mango (1 medium)
McDonald's Apple Juice Box (1)
Mott's cinnamon applesauce or
strawberry applesauce
(1 snack size)
Nectarine (2 medium)
Orange (2 medium)
Orange juice (1 cup)
Papaya (2 cups, cubed)
Pea pods (1½ cups)
Peach (2 medium)
Pear, green (2 small)
Pepino melon (2 cups,
cubed)
Persimmon (4)
Pickles (4 large)
Pineapple, canned in juice
(⅔ cup)
Pineapple juice (1 cup)
Plum (3 medium)
Pomegranate (Chinese Apple),
(1 medium)
Prickly pear (2 medium)
Prunes/dried plums (3)
Prune juice (⅔ cup)
Raisins (30)
Rhubarb, sweetened
(1 cup)
Raspberries (1½ cups)
Strawberries (2 cups)
Tangerine (4 small)

Vegetable juice, low sodium
(2 cups)
Watermelon (2 cups cubed)

SWEET TOOTH

Angel food cake (2-ounce slice)
Baker's Breakfast Cookie® (1)
Brownie (1)
Butterscotch (4 pieces)
Candy corn (20 pieces)
Chocolate-covered almonds
(7)
Fudge (1 ounce)
Gelatin (½ cup)
Graham crackers, 2½-inch
squares (3)
Granola bar, low-fat (1)
Gumdrops (1 ounce)
Healthy Choice: Novelties Low-
Fat Fudge Bar (1)
Healthy Choice: Novelties Low-
Fat Strawberry & Cream (1)
Heath bar, snack size (1)
Hershey's Bites Reese's Peanut
Butter (7)
Hershey's Bites Heath Toffee
(7)
Hershey's Bites Kit Kat Wafers
(8)
Hershey's Bites Mini Rolo
Caramels (9)
Hershey's Bites Mr. Goodbar
Chocolate (11)
Hershey's Bites York
Peppermint Pattie (9)
Hershey's Bites White
Chocolate Pretzels (11)
Hershey's Kisses (4)
Hershey's Miniature Bar, any
flavor (2)
Hershey's Miniature Nut Love,
any flavor (2)

Hershey's Sweet Escapes
(1 bar, any kind)
Kellogg's Cocoa Rice Krispies
Bar (1)
Kit Kat (2-piece bar)
Kudos with M&M's granola
bar (1)
McDonald's Apple Dippers with
Low-Fat Caramel Dip
M&M's plain (1 mini bag)
M&M's Peanut, fun size
(1 bag)
M&M's Peanut Butter, fun size
(1 bag)
Milky Way Dark, fun size (1)
Nature Valley Granola Bar, all
flavors (1 bar)
No Pudge! Fat-Free Fudge
Brownie (2-inch square)
PayDay, snack size (1)
Peanut brittle (1 ounce)
Popsicle Fudgesicle Bar (1)
Pound cake (1-ounce slice)
Pria Bar, all flavors,
(1 bar)
Pudding cup, fat-free (1)
Reese's Peanut Butter Cup
(1 snack size)
See's lollipop, any flavor (1)
Sherbet (½ cup)
Skinny Cow Fat Free Fudge
Bar (1)
Skinny Cow Low Fat Ice Cream
Sandwich (½)
Stretch Island Fruit Leather,
any flavor (2)
Tofutti (¼ cup)
Whoppers malted milk balls (9)
Yogurt, frozen, low-fat or non-
fat (½ cup)
Yogurt, low-fat or nonfat
(6 ounces)

CRUNCHY/SALTY

Almonds (12)
Baked! Cheetos Crunchy (1 small bag)
Breadsticks, 4 inches (2)
Cashews (12)
Cheez-It Twisterz (12)
Chips, baked, tortilla or potato (¾ ounce or 15–20 chips)
Genisoy Soy Crisps (25)
Goldfish crackers, Four Cheese (25)
Handi-Snacks, Mister Salty Pretzels 'n Cheese (1 pack)
Jolly Time Minis Healthy Pop Butter Flavor (1 bag)
Melba toast (4 slices)
Nabisco Ritz Chips, Cheddar (10 chips)
Nabisco Ritz Chips, Regular (10 chips)
Nabisco Ritz Chips, Sour Cream & Onion (10 chips)
Orville Redenbacher's Popcorn Mini Cakes, all flavors (10 cakes)
Oyster crackers (24)
Peanuts (20)
Pecans (8 halves)
Popcorn, air popped (3 cups)
Potato chips, fat-free (15–20)
Pretzels (3¼ ounces)
Pringles Reduced Fat Original, 8 pack (1 pack)
Pumpkin seeds (⅓ cup)
Quaker Quakes, Cheddar Cheese (20)
Quaker Quakes, Nacho Cheese (20)
Quaker Quakes, BBQ (20)
Rice cakes (2)
Saltine crackers (6)
Sargento, Cheese Dip & Cheddar Sticks snacks (1 pack)
Sesame seeds (2 tablespoons)

Soda crackers (4)
String cheese (1)
Sunflower seeds (2 tablespoons)
Tortilla chips, fat free (15–20)
Trader Joe's Low-Fat Rice Crisps, Caramel (14 crisps)
Trader Joe's Low-Fat White Cheddar Corn Crisps (20 crisps)
Uncle Sam Cereal (½ cup dry)
Whole grain crackers (2–5)

SNACK PACKS

Nabisco 100-Calorie Pack, Chips Ahoy Thin Crisps (1 bag)
Nabisco 100-Calorie Pack, Kraft Cheese Nips thin crisps (1 bag)
Nabisco 100-Calorie Pack, Oreo thin crisps (1 bag)
Nabisco 100-Calorie Pack, Wheat Thins minis (1 bag)
Nabisco 100-Calorie Pack, Honey Maid Cinnamon thin crisps (1 bag)
Nabisco 100-Calorie Pack, Ritz Snack Mix (1 bag)

COFFEE HOUSE

Starbucks® Beverages
Grande Nonfat Cappuccino
Grande Nonfat Café Latte
Grande Shaken Iced Coffee
Grande Tazo Iced Tea (black or passion)
Tall Nonfat Sugar-Free Vanilla Latte
Tall Nonfat Sugar-Free Iced Vanilla Latte
Tall Tazo Tea Lemonade

Starbucks Snacks
Starbucks has some great snacks that you can enjoy with a regular coffee, complete with skim milk and Splenda. Remember to have only one of these snacks.
Chocolate Hazelnut Biscotti
Vanilla Almond Biscotti
Madeleine

Coffee Bean & Tea Leaf
Café Mocha with no-sugar-added/fat-free powder, 12 ounces
Café Vanilla with no-sugar-added/fat-free powder, 12 ounces
Chai Iced Blended with no-sugar-added/fat-free powder, 12 ounces
Extreme Ice Blended with no-sugar-added/fat-free powder, 12 ounces
Iced Café Latte with whole milk, 16 ounces
Iced Cappuccino with whole milk, 16 ounces
Iced Chai Tea Latte with no-sugar-added/fat-free powder, 24 ounces
Iced Mocha Latte with no-sugar-added/fat-free powder, 16 ounces
Iced Vanilla Latte with no-sugar-added/fat-free powder, 16 ounces
Nonfat Iced Café Latte, 24 ounces
Nonfat Cappuccino, single
Nonfat Café Latte, 12 ounces
Nonfat Iced Cappuccino, 24 ounces

Gas Station Gourmet
We've all been there: you're stuck on the road and it's time for your next snack. This section includes a list of food items commonly found at ampm, 7-Eleven, Circle K, or whichever gas station mini-mart you may be passing by. Use this list to help you make smart selections when you're car-bound.

Almonds (12)
Baked! Cheetos Crunchy (1 small bag)
Candy corn (20 pieces)
Cashews (12)
Chocolate-covered almonds (7)
Fruit cocktail (1 cup)
Granola bar, low-fat (1)
Graham crackers, 2½ inch squares (3)
Grapefruit juice (1 cup)
Gumdrops (1 ounce)
Handi-Snacks, Mister Salty Pretzels 'n Cheese (1 pack)
Hershey's Kisses (4)
Kit Kat (2-piece bar)
Nature Valley Granola Bar, all flavors (1 bar)
Orange juice (1 cup)
Peanuts (20)
Pineapple juice (1 cup)
Popcorn, air-popped (3 cups)
Potato chips, fat-free (15–20)
Pretzels (3¼ ounces)
Pudding cup, fat-free (1)
Pumpkin seeds (⅓ cup)
Raisins (30)
Rice cakes (2)
Saltine crackers (6)
String cheese (1)
Tortilla chips, fat free (15–20)
Vegetable juice, low-sodium (2 cups)
Whoppers malted milk balls (9)

Chapter 14
DESSERTS

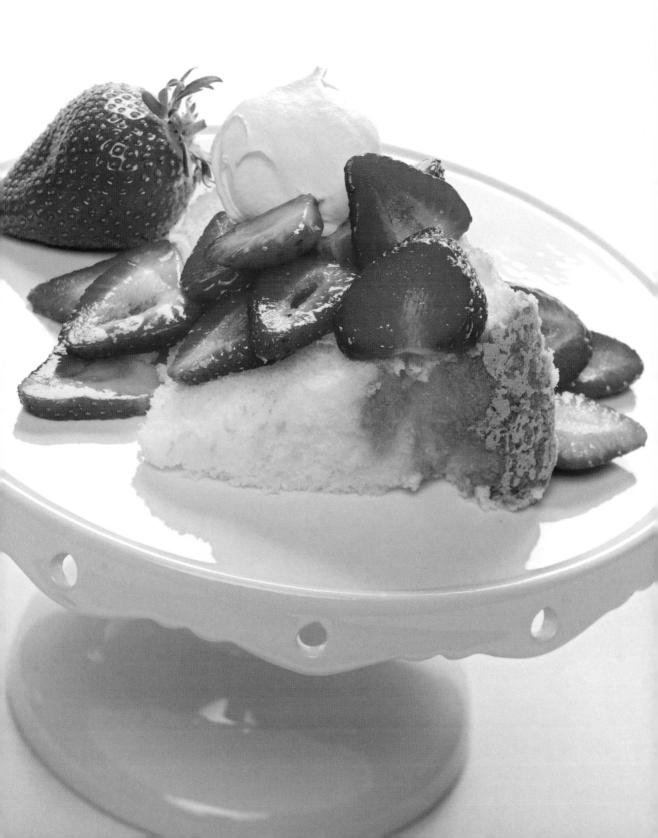

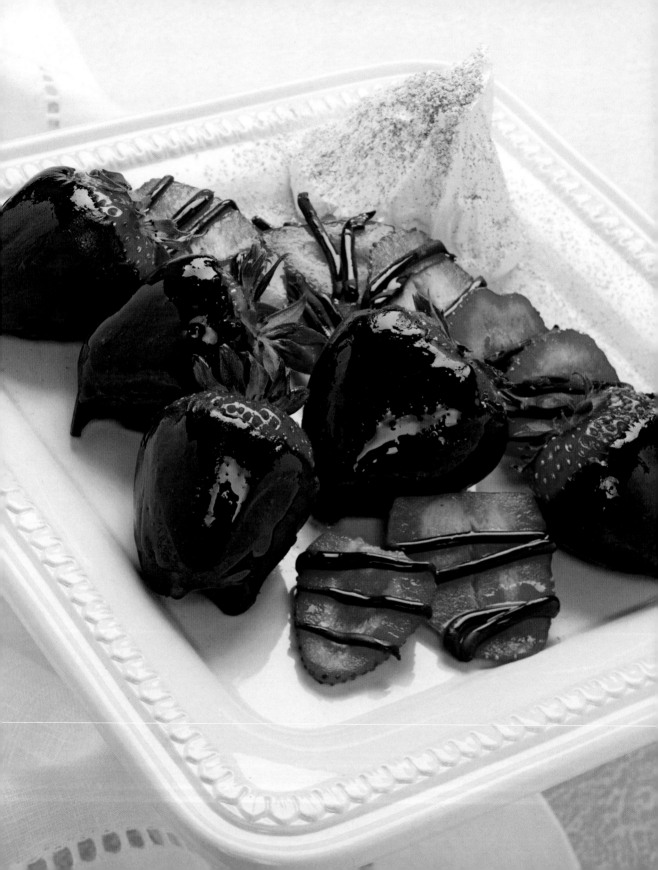

CHOCOLATE-COVERED STRAWBERRIES

Chocolate-covered strawberries and cream—you'll forget you're on a diet when you indulge in this luscious concoction.

MAKES 4 SERVINGS

1½ ounces semisweet chocolate chips
12 strawberries, sliced
4 tablespoons nonfat whipped topping

Place the chocolate chips in a small microwave-safe bowl and microwave until melted, 20 seconds, stirring frequently. Place the strawberries on a platter and drizzle with the melted chocolate. Top with the whipped topping and serve.

LADYFINGER PARFAIT

Bright blue blueberries turn this simple vanilla yogurt parfait into an elegant ending to any dinner.

MAKES 4 SERVINGS

4 ladyfingers
1 cup fat-free vanilla frozen yogurt
½ cup blueberries

Layer one ladyfinger, ¼ cup frozen yogurt, and 2 tablespoons blueberries in each of four small glasses. Serve.

RICE PUDDING IN PHYLLO CRUST

Phyllo, also called fillo, dough is a thin, flaky pastry that is often used in Mediterranean desserts and casseroles. Frozen phyllo dough is available in the frozen pastry section of most supermarkets.

MAKES 4 SERVINGS

Cooking spray
2 sheets of phyllo dough, thawed
2 prepared single-serving nonfat rice puddings
2 tablespoons nonfat whipped topping
1 teaspoon cinnamon

1.   Preheat the oven to 400°F.

2. Spray a muffin tin with cooking spray.

3. Slice the phyllo sheets in quarters and line the muffin cups with two layers. Spray the top of each sheet with cooking spray.

4. Bake until just browned, 4 minutes.

5. Carefully remove the phyllo cups from the muffin pan and place on a plate.

6. Fill each cup with one-fourth of the rice pudding, top with the whipped topping, sprinkle with cinnamon, and serve.

JELL-O PARFAIT

Simple, quick, and easy to make, this colorful dessert combination makes a stunning picture on your dining room table.

MAKES 4 SERVINGS

4 prepared sugar-free Jell-O® cups, any flavor
1 medium banana, sliced
2 prepared fat-free vanilla pudding cups

In each of four clear glasses, layer one-fourth of the Jell-O®, one-fourth of the banana slices, and one-fourth of the pudding and serve.

STRAWBERRY SHORTCAKE

You can enjoy this refreshing summery dessert any time of year. If straw-berries are out of season, substitute unsweetened frozen berries.

MAKES 4 SERVINGS

2 slices (⅛ of cake each) store-bought angel food cake, sliced in half
1 cup thinly sliced strawberries
4 tablespoons nonfat whipped topping
1 teaspoon powdered sugar

Place a half slice of angel food cake on each of four plates. Top with strawberries and whipped topping. Sprinkle with powdered sugar and serve.

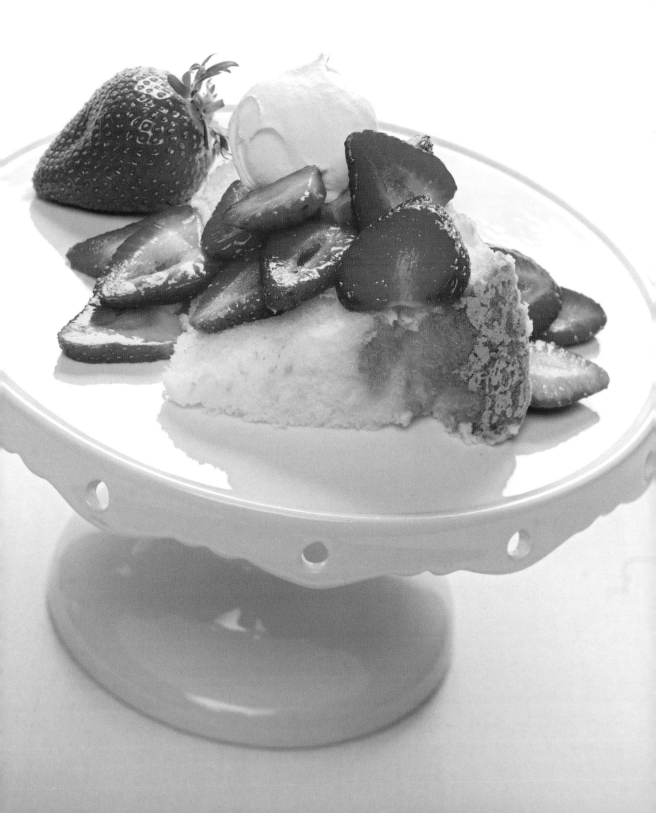

FROSTED CAPPUCCINO SHAKE

Feeling like a lift? Try this chilled hazelnut cappuccino. It has all the caffeine and flavor of your favorite coffeehouse specialty but with a fraction of the fat and calories.

MAKES 4 SERVINGS

2 cups prepared, chilled hazelnut coffee
2 cups skim milk
1 teaspoon chocolate extract
4 packets artificial sweetener
2 tablespoons nonfat whipped topping
2 teaspoons cocoa powder

1. Combine coffee, milk, chocolate extract, and artificial sweetener in a bowl and whisk until frothy.

2. Fill four tall glasses with ice and pour coffee mixture evenly in each.

3. Spoon on the whipped topping, dust with cocoa powder, and serve.

FROZEN BANANA ICE CREAM

An alternative to dairy ice cream, this frozen banana concoction is great for vegans and lactose-intolerant individuals.

MAKES 4 SERVINGS

2 large frozen bananas, peeled and diced
2 tablespoons water
½ cup berries

1. Combine the bananas and water in a mini food processor and blend until smooth.

2. Divide among four bowls and garnish each with 2 tablespoons berries.

APRICOT-ALMOND MERINGUE SANDWICH COOKIES

Meringue cookies are made of egg whites that are beaten until stiff peaks form. Sweet, light, crisp, and delicious, you'll forget that these cookies are fat-free.

4 store-bought meringue cookies
4 teaspoon all-fruit apricot spread
¼ teaspoon almond extract
¼ cup nonfat whipped topping

1. With a serrated knife, carefully slice each cookie in half, like a hamburger bun, and hollow out the inside.

2. Add 1 teaspoon of the fruit spread to the bottom half of each cookie.

3. Stir the almond extract into the whipped topping and add 1 tablespoon to each cookie bottom.

4. Sandwich the top half of the cookie onto the bottom and serve.

Variations

Chocolate-Cherry Meringue Sandwich Cookies: use cherry fruit spread and add 1 teaspoon cocoa powder to the whipped topping.

Vanilla-Orange Meringue Sandwich Cookies: use orange fruit spread and add ¼ teaspoon vanilla extract to the whipped topping.

Minted Strawberry Meringue Sandwich Cookies: use strawberry fruit spread and add ¼ teaspoon peppermint extract to the whipped topping.

Brandied Plum Meringue Sandwich Cookies: use plum fruit spread and add ¼ teaspoon brandy extract to the whipped topping.

APPLE CUPS

This is another dish that I made with Emeril on his show. This dessert is a bit of a splurge—it has 100 calories per serving instead of 50. Serve this beautiful apple compote in petal-like phyllo cups to company for a show-stopping presentation.

3 medium Granny Smith apples, peeled and thinly sliced
½ teaspoon stevia
½ teaspoon lemon zest
½ teaspoon orange zest
2 tablespoons orange juice
2 tablespoons water
1 teaspoon cinnamon
Pinch freshly grated nutmeg
Cooking spray
3 sheets phyllo dough, thawed

1. Preheat oven to 350°F.

2. In a medium saucepan over medium heat, combine apples, stevia, zests, orange juice, water, cinnamon and nutmeg. Cook until apples begin to break down, 10 minutes.

3. Meanwhile, place three sheets phyllo on cutting board and cut into 5-inch squares.

4. Place one square on a work surface and spray with cooking spray. Place a second square over the first, turning so the corners are not aligned. Spray again with cooking spray. Add a third layer using the same method and spray one more time with cooking spray.

5. Lightly coat a silicone muffin pan with cooking spray and press the center of the squares into the muffin cups.

6. Spoon the warm apple mixture into the center of each cup, distributing evenly in the four cups. Bake for 10 to 12 minutes or until the outer edges of the cups are lightly browned.

7. Serve each person one apple cup.

MELON JELL-O

Using honeydew melon instead of a bowl to hold the Jell-O® while it cools in the fridge not only saves on dishwashing, it also adds flavor.

MAKES 4 SERVINGS

One 3-ounce package sugar-free lime Jell-O®
½ honeydew melon, cleaned of seeds and pulp
2 tablespoons nonfat whipped topping

1. Add the Jell-O powder to a small bowl and add 1 cup boiling water. Stir to dissolve. Let the Jell-O cool slightly.

2. Cut a thin slice from the bottom of the honeydew half to stabilize it.

3. Pour the Jell-O into the melon, taking care not to overfill. Cover with plastic wrap and chill until set in refrigerator (refrigerate leftover Jell-O mixture for another dessert or snack).

4. When the Jell-O is completely set, serve the melon family-style, topped with whipped topping.

VANILLA PUDDING WITH BANANA

This simple, soft comfort food is similar to banana cream pie.

MAKES 4 SERVINGS

2 prepared individual fat-free vanilla pudding cups
1 banana, thinly sliced
1 tablespoon graham cracker crumbs

In four small cups, layer the banana slices and then the pudding. Sprinkle with graham cracker crumbs and serve.

APPLE STRUDEL

The aroma of apple pie will fill your kitchen when you bake this tasty, healthy version of apple strudel.

MAKES 4 SERVINGS

Cooking spray
2 sheets phyllo dough, thawed
1 large apple, peeled, cored, and thinly sliced
2 packets artificial sweetener
2 teaspoons cinnamon

1. Preheat the oven to 400°F.

2. Spray a baking sheet with cooking spray and lay one sheet of phyllo dough on it. Spray the phyllo with cooking spray, top with the second sheet of phyllo, and spray again.

3. Layer the apple, artificial sweetener, and cinnamon on the phyllo and roll into a log. Lay seam-side down and fold in the ends. Spray the outside of the log with cooking spray and cut 4 angled slashes through the top.

4. Bake until golden brown, 6 to 8 minutes.

5. Slice the strudel into four equal portions and serve.

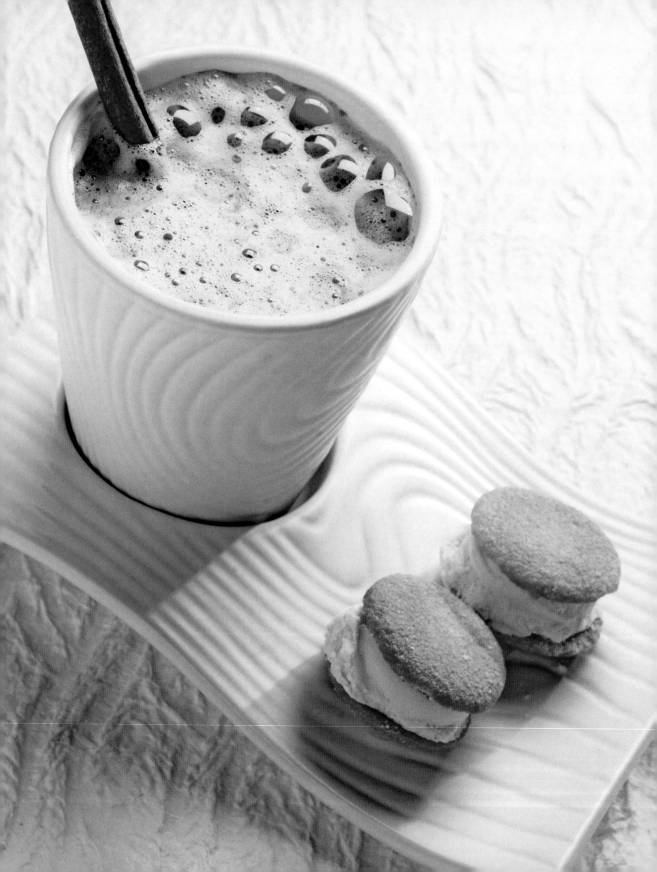

MINI ICE CREAM SANDWICH

You can't go wrong with an ice cream sandwich. Choose a nonfat variety of vanilla, chocolate, or strawberry ice cream to make this delectable dessert.

MAKES 4 SERVINGS

16 reduced-fat Nilla® wafers
1 cup fat-free vanilla ice cream, softened

1. Scoop 2 tablespoons of ice cream on each of 8 Nilla wafers, top with the remaining cookies.

2. Serve each person four ice cream sandwiches.

CINNAMON SUGAR POPCORN

Watching a movie tonight? Enjoy an alternative to traditional popcorn with this sweetened version of the old standard.

MAKES 4 SERVINGS

4 packets artificial sweetener
1 tablespoon brown sugar
2 teaspoons cinnamon
4 cups air-popped popcorn
Cooking spray

Stir together artificial sweetener, sugar, and cinnamon in a small bowl. Spray the popcorn with cooking spray. Sprinkle the cinnamon-sugar mixture on the popcorn and serve.

YOGURT PARFAIT

This is a great dish to make with children. If your kids like to help you in the kitchen, let them arrange the layers of this colorful yogurt parfait.

MAKES 4 SERVINGS

2 cups low-fat vanilla yogurt
1½ cups mixed berries (thawed if frozen)
2 tablespoons fat-free whipped topping

Layer the yogurt, mixed berries, and whipped topping in four small cups. Serve.

NEED EVEN FASTER 50-CALORIE DESSERTS? TRY THESE:

3 Musketeers minis (2)

Animal crackers (4)

Caramel (2 ½-ounce pieces)

Cheese slice, reduced-calorie (1 ounce)

Chocolate chips (½ tablespoon)

Chocolate-coated mints (4)

Cookie, butter (1)

Cookie, fat-free (1 small)

Cookie, fortune (1)

Corn cake (1)

Cranberry sauce (¼ cup)

European chestnuts (1 ounce)

Frozen seedless grapes (1 cup)

Gelatin dessert, sugar-free (1)

Gingersnaps (3)

Ginkgo nuts (1 ounce or 14 medium)

Graham cracker (1 2½-inch square)

Gumdrops (2)

Hard candy (1)

Hershey's Bites Reese's Peanut Butter (4)

Hershey's Bites Heath Toffee (4)

Hershey's Bites Kit Kat Wafers (4)

Hershey's Bites Mini Rolo Caramels (5)

Hershey's Bites Mr. Goodbar Chocolate (5)

Hershey's Bites York Peppermint Pattie (5)

Hershey's Bites White Chocolate Pretzels (6)

Hershey's Hugs or Kisses (2)

Hershey's Miniature Bar, any flavor (1)

Hershey's Miniature Nut Love, any flavor (1)

Hershey's Nugget, any flavor (1)

Ice milk, vanilla (¼ cup)

Ice pop, made with water (2-ounce pop)

Jelly beans (7)

Licorice twist (1)

LifeSavers, all-fruit flavor (3)

LifeSavers, Lollipop, swirled flavor (1)

M&M's (¼ of snack-size bag)

M&M's Minis (¼ of tube)

Marshmallow (1 large)

Marshmallows, mini (¼ cup)

McDonald's Kiddie Cone

Miss Meringue cookie (1)

Nestle Crunch miniature (1)

Nestle Turtles Bite Size (1)

Nonfat ice cream (½ cup) drizzled with 1 tablespoon Hershey's chocolate syrup

Oreo cookie (1)

Popcorn, air popped (1 cup)

Popsicle ACE Juice Pops (1)

Popsicle Creamsicle Sugar-Free Pops (2)

Popsicle Mighty Magic Minis (1)

Popsicle Red, White & Blue Ice Pops (1)

Popsicle Swirlwinds Ice Pops (1)

Pretzels (½ ounce)

Prune (1)

Raisins (1 tablespoon)

Raisins, chocolate covered (10)

Reese's Peanut Butter Cup (1)

Rice Krispies Treat square (½)

Ritz Bits, peanut butter (5)

SnackWell's sandwich cookie (1)

Starburst fruit chew (3 pieces)

Stretch Island Fruit Leather, any flavor (1)

Switzer Cherry Bites (12)

Switzer Licorice Bites (12)

Teddy Grahams, honey flavor (6)

Tootsie Roll Pop, any flavor (1)

Triscuit crackers (2)

Vanilla wafers (2)

York Peppermint Pattie (1 small)

Chapter 15
COCKTAILS

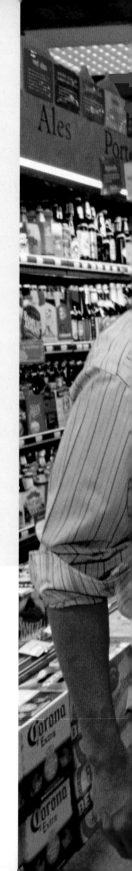

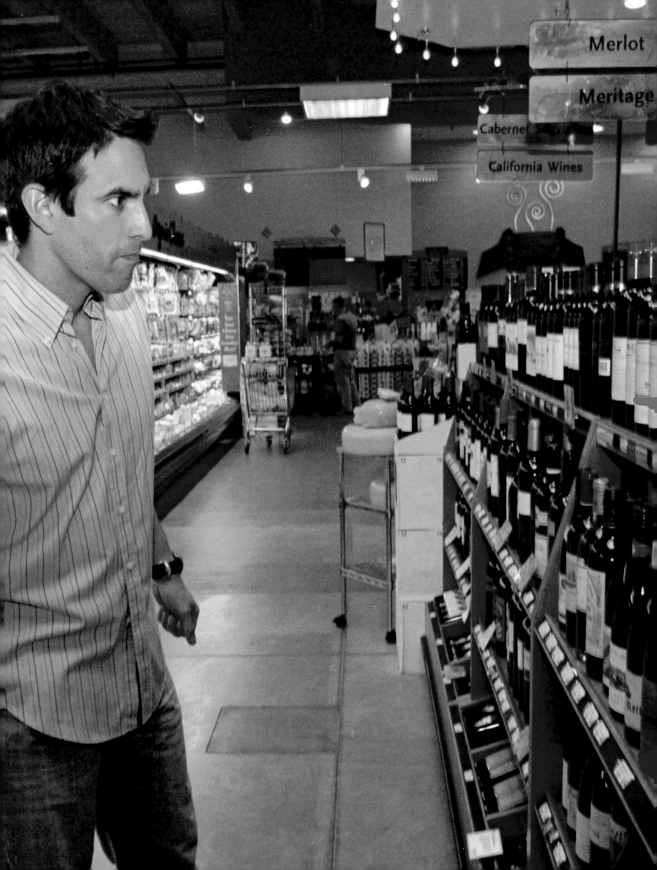

Although I don't recommend drinking too much while trying to lose weight, here's how you can indulge occasionally. Choose either option A or B below. Option A allows you to replace your evening treat with one drink and option B allows more than one drink if you follow the "drink reserve" guidelines.

Option A: If you feel like having a drink with your dinner in the evening, make it your treat, but be sure it fits the program. Here are some ideas:

1. Make a 3-Hour Diet™–approved Wine Spritzer. Check the chart on page 331 for tips on how to mix it.

2. Make a 3-Hour Diet™–approved cocktail such as a seven and seven with diet soda, or rum and Diet Coke® in place of your evening treat. These two are slightly more than 50 calories, but close enough for a thumbs-up. Check the chart on page 331 for tips on how to mix them.

Option B: If you want to drink more than offered in Option A, then use these three steps:

STEP 1: Set your drink count before you go out.

STEP 2: Burn the calories before you head out. You've got to burn extra calories in anticipation of consuming extra calories. That's the secret. See the chart on page 332 to decide how much exercise you need.

STEP 3: Enjoy yourself!

Note: Watch out for some popular favorites! A 5-ounce margarita packs a walloping 340 calories! A very cool 4-ounce cosmopolitan will add 250 calories to your day. You can have them, but you'll need to do more exercise to burn those extra calories.

Mixing the Perfect 3-Hour Diet™ — *Approved Cocktail*

The following chart contains some favorite cocktails with recipes to help you stay on the program while enjoying yourself. There are a few that stay in the 50-calorie range; you can have one of these in place of a treat in the evening. All of the others are approximately 100 calories, which is the amount burned with each of the "Burners" I've listed on page 332. Remember, a standard shot glass measures 1½ ounces.

50-CALORIE TREAT DRINKS

WINE SPRITZER . . . . .2.5 ounces wine (50 cal.)
6 ounces seltzer or Diet 7-Up® (0 cal.)

RUM AND DIET COKE® . . . . .1 ounce spiced rum (60 cal.)
4 ounces Diet Coke® (0 cal.)
Twist of lime (freebie)

SEVEN & DIET SEVEN. . . . . 1 ounce whiskey (60 cal.)
8 ounces diet lemon-lime soda (0 cal.)
Twist of lime (freebie)

CHERRY BOMB VODKA. . . . . . . 1 ounce Red Cherry vodka (60 cal.)
6 ounces Diet Cherry Coke® (0 cal.)

DIET VODKA TONIC. . . . . 1 ounce vodka (60 cal.)
6 ounces diet tonic (0 cal.)
Twist of lime (freebie)

100-CALORIE COCKTAILS

VODKA TONIC . . . . 1 ounce vodka (60 cal.)
4 ounces tonic (40 cal.)
Twist of lime (freebie)

BLOODY MARY. . . . . .1.5 ounces vodka (90 cal.)
4 ounces/.5 cup tomato juice (20 cal.)
Lime twist, dash Tabasco®, dash pepper, dash Worcestershire (freebies)
1 celery stick (freebie)

LIGHT BEER— they vary, check the label . . 12 ounces (one regular size can or bottle)

Miller Lite, Amstel Light, Aspen Edge,
Natural Light, Michelob Ultra . . . . 95 cal
Coors Light . . . . 102 cal
Bud Light, Bud Ice Light, Busch Light . . . . 110 cal

RED OR WHITE WINE . . . . 5 ounces (100 cal.)
(no port/dessert wine)

GIN AND TONIC . . . . 1 ounce gin (60 cal.)
4 ounces tonic (40 cal.)
Twist of lime (freebie)

GIMLET .1.5 ounces gin or vodka (90 cal.)
.5 ounce sweetened lime juice (4 cal.)
Twist of lime (freebie)

BLOODY MARIA .1.5 ounce tequila (90 cal.)
4 ounces/.5 cup tomato juice (20 cal.)
Lemon twist, dash Tabasco®, dash salt (freebies)

RUM AND COKE . . . . .1 ounce spiced rum (60 cal.)
4 ounces Coca-Cola® (48 cal.)
Twist of lime (freebie)

SEVEN & SEVEN. . . . . 1 ounce whiskey (60 cal.)
2 ounces reg. lemon-lime soda (28 cal.)
6 ounces diet lemon-lime soda (0 cal.)
Twist of lime (freebie)

VODKA & DIET VANILLA COKE® . . . . .1.5 ounces vodka (90 cal.)
8 ounces Diet Vanilla Coke® (0 cal.)

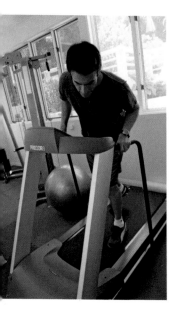

How to Create the Drink Reserve

Below you'll find some activities to help you burn off those 100-calorie cocktails. Remember, you have to multiply how long you do the activity by how many drinks you plan to have. If you decide to splurge on a higher-calorie drink, you'll have to exercise more to balance it out.

THE BURNERS	DURATION
(each one creates a 100-calorie reserve)	
Walking 3 mph	19 minutes
Jogging 5 mph	11 minutes
Energetic dancing	14 minutes
Active aerobics	12 minutes
Biking	12 minutes
Steady swimming	11 minutes
Vigorous housecleaning (floor scrubbing, vacuuming, sweeping)	20 minutes
Gardening (raking, mowing, squatting to pull weeds)	15 minutes
Washing car	20 minutes
Active sex	20 minutes

SPECIAL THANKS

Recipes developed in association with the School of Nutrition and Exercise Science at Bastyr University: At the heart of natural medicine.

Egg Sandwich (page 52)

Veggie Sausage and Egg Sandwich (page 56)

Oats with Turkey Bacon (page 75)

Almond Butter and Banana Toast (page 80)

Egg Breakfast Burrito (page 57)

Cereal with Milk and Cottage Cheese (page 41)

Scrambled Eggs with English Muffins (page 58)

Breakfast Ham and Cheese (page 78)

Toast with Almond Butter and Cottage Cheese (page 82)

Muesli and Fruit (page 85)

Breakfast Tacos (page 61)

Breakfast Burrito (page 80)

Waffles with Almond Butter (page 83)

Apples, Walnuts, and Yogurt (page 92)

Orange and Banana Smoothie (page 96)

Breakfast Smoothie (page 96)

Turkey Sausage Pasta with Kale (page 101)

Broiled Salmon and Brussels Sprouts (page 150)

Salmon and Brown Rice (page 153)

Cajun Catfish with Sautéed Greens (page 154)

White Fish and Potatoes (page 158)

Chili and Potatoes (page 168)

Potstickers, Beans, and Greens (page 169)

Turkey Sandwich with Coleslaw (page 220)

Pork Chops with Squash Soup (page 203)

Tuna Sandwich and Tomato Soup (page 232)

Turkey Tortilla Wrap (page 239)

Salmon Burgers and Sugar Snap Peas (page 242)

Turkey and Cranberry Sandwich (page 245)

Chicken and Cranberry Salad (page 252)

Spinach Beet Salad (page 256)

Salmon Salad (page 258)

Chicken Waldorf Salad (page 261)

Gardenburgers with Vegetable Crudités (page 273)

Vegetarian Chili (page 272)

Burrito and Greens (page 274)

Chickpea Vegetable Curry (page 279)

Franks and Beans (page 280)

Mediterranean Pita (page 284)

Miso Soup with Soba Noodles (page 283)

INDEX